Deep Tissue Massage

Art Riggs presents a masterful blend of technical information and insightful practical theory. *Deep Tissue Massage* is well organized, clearly written, and supported by high-quality instructional photographs and anatomical drawings. This book will be of great use for a range of bodyworkers, from massage therapists to sophisticated medical practitioners.

—HELEN JAMES, PROFESSOR EMERITA PHYSICAL THERAPY,
CALIFORNIA STATE UNIVERSITY, FRESNO

Art Riggs has dedicated himself for over a decade to sharing his knowledge and wisdom of the body. We highly recommend this book for massage students and health professionals alike.

—PAULETTE AND RICHARD BERGESS, DIRECTORS,
THE SAN FRANCISCO SCHOOL OF MASSAGE

Deep Tissue Massage

A Visual Guide to Techniques

Revised Edition

Art Riggs

Certified Advanced Rolfer, CMT

Foreword by Thomas W. Myers

North Atlantic Books
Berkeley, California

Published by
North Atlantic Books
P.O. Box 12327
Berkeley, California 94712

Photographs by David Booth
Cover design by Claudia Smelser
Book design by Paula Morrison
Printed in the United States of America

The author gratefully acknowledges permission from Williams and Wilkins for the rights to reproduce the anatomical drawing in this book, taken from *Myofascial Pain and Dysfunction: The Trigger Point Manual, Volumes I and II, 1992*, by Travell and Simons. I very highly recommend the wonderful cadaver dissection video series, *The Video Atlas of Human Anatomy*, also distributed by Williams and Wilkins.

Deep Tissue Massage: A Visual Guide to Techniques is sponsored by the Society for the Study of Native Arts and Sciences, a nonprofit educational corporation whose goals are to develop an educational and crosscultural perspective linking various scientific, social, and artistic fields; to nurture a holistic view of arts, sciences, humanities, and healing; and to publish and distribute literature on the relationship of mind, body, and nature.

North Atlantic Books' publications are available through most bookstores. For further information, call 800-337-2665 or visit our website at www.northatlanticbooks.com. Substantial discounts on bulk quantities are available to corporations, professional associations, and other organizations. For details and discount information, contact our special sales department.

Library of Congress Cataloging-in-Publication Data

Riggs, Art.
    Deep tissue massage : a visual guide to techniques / Art Riggs ; foreword by Thomas W. Myers. — Rev. ed.
        p. ; cm.
    Includes bibliographical references and index.
    ISBN 978-1-55643-650-5 (pbk.)
        1. Massage therapy. 2. Massage therapy—Atlases. I. Title.
        [DNLM: 1. Massage—methods—Atlases. WE 17 R569d 2007]
    RM721 R544 2007
    615.8'22—dc22
                                                                2007009953

7 8 9 10 11 12 13 14 UNITED 14 13 12 11 10 09 08 07

I feel blessed to have been chosen by a profession where I can continue learning new skills until the day I can no longer work.

—Helen "Jimmer" James, a Rolfing Teacher

Acknowledgments

IT IS A DAUNTING TASK TO NAME ALL THOSE who have molded me into the bodyworker that am today and who have contributed to my attempts to express some of what I know in this book. Properly expressing my gratitude would be as difficult as attempting to perform an extensive full-body Deep Tissue Massage in fifteen minutes. Rather than inadvertently omitting the name of a dear friend or teacher, except for several names of particular significance, I will acknowledge a few broad groups to whom I am deeply thankful. I hope that all of my guides will recognize my gratitude to them in my broad descriptions.

This book would never have been written without the encouragement and exhortations of my good friend, fellow Rolfer®, and distinguished teacher, Michael Stanborough. For several years I used his excellent manual, *Myofascial Release: An Illustrative and Photographic Manual* as the text in my massage classes. With Michael's encouragement and blessings, and using his book as a model, I wrote a manual that more closely followed the curriculum of my classes. This manual evolved into the present edition of *Deep Tissue Massage: A Visual Guide To Techniques*.

To all my teachers, particularly those at the Rolf Institute, I offer my heartfelt thanks for the generous sharing of your expertise and philosophies. You gave your knowledge with love—not doling it out as a commodity, and you asked nothing in return. With your patience and lack of judgment, you freed me to demonstrate my ignorance and removed the insecurity that so often accompanies the acquisition of knowledge. I hope that I can embody your wisdom both in my work and in my teaching.

Most of us have one teacher who transcends the ordinary and becomes a mentor, and I would like to thank Michael Salveson for his continued patient attempts at my edification over the years. He transformed bodywork from rote procedure to a complex, rewarding, and fun game. Not a day goes by that I do not conjure up Michael and other teachers as apparitions, standing over my shoulder, offering suggestions on how to help deal with some particular issue related to a client. Yes Michael, I promise to slow down and listen to what the client's tissue is telling me.

To my clients, thank you for making my work so rewarding. For working with me to achieve your goals rather than expecting to be magically transformed without your participation. Without my love for my work and clients, I would never have the desire to share my knowledge and passion for this profession with a wider audience in a manual such as this one.

Much gratitude to those who have helped me with their suggestions for the book: for constructive criticisms as well as support. To my photographer, David Booth for his wonderful pictures and to my copyeditor, Michele Chase, I extend my sincerest apologetic thanks for good naturedly putting up with my nit-picking and also for forcing me to listen to your nit-picking when I didn't want to. I also wish to thank Paula Morrison for her artistic expertise in the difficult job of designing a clear and cohesive book with hundreds of photographs and anatomical drawings. Thanks are also owed to my model, Dena Lofthus.

Most of all, I thank my students over the years. I appreciate your openness to learning and your enthusiasm. I assure you that the learning has been reciprocal. This book is for you.

Contents

List of Figures

Chapter Three

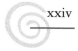

Chapter Six

Foreword

Our time presents two conflicting but contemporaneous currents: On the one hand, our culture is in general becoming increasingly alienated from its own bodily experience. We are ever more sedentary and obese as we spend more time in chairs in front of the heady temptation of TV's, computers, and video games. Physical education, its standard repetitious fare outdated in any case, becomes a vanishingly small part of our children's education. A barrage of advertising and audio-visual stimulation leaves us out of touch with our true inner feelings and intuitions.

At the same time, however, sports records continue to be broken with astonishing feats of athleticism unknown from earlier times, and more well-prepared and technologically equipped bodies are bravely expanding our reach into the *Ultima Thule*—in space, the oceans, and the most forbidding terrain of our planet, where new equipment makes it possible and even comfortable to boldly go where no one yet has been. And finally, a small group of therapists and teachers are enjoying a renaissance in what could be called the "somatic arts," but is generally grouped these days under the name "massage."

Over the last half century, massage has grown from a tiny minority of practitioners giving relaxational massage to a vitally expanding industry encompassing a wide variety of methods and approaches—all of which share direct contact with the body, and all of which value and validate the sensations and feelings which arise from our somatic self. These approaches include more esoteric energetic approaches such as cranial and Polarity, sheer laying on of hands as in Therapeutic Touch, and more prosaic but extremely effective approaches to sports injury recovery and prevention, as well as performance enhancement. We have seen the rise of orthopedic massage and trigger-point work, which can effectively deal with sub-clinical pains and strains otherwise beyond the scope of standard medical practice. Infant and perinatal massage, as well as pre– and post-operative cancer massage have likewise expanded the role that hands-on therapy can provide to those within the medical system. The closely related field of movement therapy has bloomed into the culture with yoga, Pilates, the Alexander Technique, Feldenkrais, and a host of related arts.

The book you hold in your hand is a contribution to what is for me a very exciting approach within this general renaissance—an approach I prefer to call Spatial Medicine. What can you change—in terms of posture, structure, function, and affect—by changing the spatial relationships within the body? Over the thirty years of my association with Rolfing and other forms of structural work, we in this field have seen some remarkable results (though as yet anecdotal—research awaits!) in terms of stress reduction, pain cessation, trauma recovery, restoration of movement range and function, postural change, and results on a psychosomatic level (attitude) that attest to the mind-body interaction.

While many of the diverse methods within the somatic realm are effective, there is something uniquely immediate about direct, deep, slow contact with what Robert Schleip, Ph.D., termed the "neuro-myofascial web." Art Riggs' *Deep Tissue Massage,* in the form of this book and the accompanying set of DVDs, provides a guide into the specifics of this form of Spatial Medicine, and a very effective and thorough one at that. No book substitutes for one-on-one class instruction, but Art Riggs makes a very good attempt at it by including all the caveats, contraindications, and the sometimes surprising aspects of effective touch. An extensive section on body use and client placement, the nature of Deep Tissue strokes, and notes on pain and touch refinement all set a context for the meticulous technique sections, organized first regionally, and then according to common complaints. A final section of the book attends to single– and multi-session strategies, and how to market Deep Tissue work to your clients. With the proviso that no book can convey the art of working with each individual pattern in an integrated way, Art Riggs has done a fine job of setting you up with all the tools necessary to begin the process of learning that elusive and not-easily-grasped skill.

In conjunction with the excellent DVDs, which are keyed to this book, Art Riggs has done a careful job of showing the new or experienced practitioner what to do, how to do it, and—equally importantly—how not to do it, to avoid injury to either the client or the practitioner. I have been pleased to recommend this book and DVD combination to my students since it was initially issued, and happy to be asked to provide a foreword to this second edition.

This handbook speaks to both the daily practicalities of getting the work done—the anatomy, the placement of the therapist's body and hands, and the intended result for the client—but it also attends to the surrounding subtler issues, making sure the work gets done in the right context, bringing about the best results for all concerned. An important addition for any beginning structural therapist, it will also serve those who wish to be reminded of the fundamentals of our art.

The plasticity of the neuro-myofascial web is the fundamental premise of Spatial Medicine. The changes and transformations that we have seen using these types of Deep Tissue techniques—applied intelligently, sensitively, and sequentially—can produce a higher level of functioning that indicates just how malleable the human body is, even in the later decades of life. While relief of pain is both a noble and practical goal, the results of this work can sometimes transcend "fixing a problem" to reach a developmental transformation that points to an exciting future for this field and for the sincere practitioners who labor within it. To undertake a career in deep manual therapy is to embark on an exciting journey of discovery, one in which you will seldom be bored, often challenged, and continually rewarded with the best that a healing interaction has to offer—a combination of gratitude, humility, and affirmation that is, according to Saint Francis, good for the soul.

Thomas W. Myers
Author of *Anatomy Trains*

Preface to the 2007 Edition

D RAMATIC CHANGES IN THE FIELD OF MASSAGE have taken place in the short time since the first printing of *Deep Tissue Massage* five years ago. Not only has relaxation-based massage expanded exponentially each year, both in the number of practitioners and in acceptance by the general population, but also "therapeutic" bodywork is increasingly accepted by both the public and the medical profession as an extremely effective treatment for a variety of conditions (see pages 156–157 for a summary of a recent study on this topic). No longer the sphere of counterculture alternative healers, massage is increasingly prescribed by doctors for their patients, and insurance companies are frequently covering massage because they are learning that not only is massage effective, but it also saves them money as an effective choice of treatment.

Most of the changes taking place are positive, but the industry is experiencing growing pains, seen, for instance, in licensing regulations or continuing education requirements that often have little to do with the welfare of either clients or practitioners. States, local municipalities, large massage organizations, and competing schools are vying for power and for students. Sadly, the almighty dollar is often the motivating force behind arbitrary requirements for training and continuing education. These do not necessarily insure that therapists are becoming more accomplished in their work, especially in the absence of consensus about what constitutes various levels of skill or competence.

Although schools offer excellent continuing education programs, many of these are extensive and expensive programs of many hundreds of hours, which are increasingly technical, specialized, and downright intimidating for some. Many massage practitioners are feeling pressured to drastically alter the work they love in order to "keep up" with these new developments. Most therapists applying for jobs at spas, chiropractors' offices, and other venues are now required to have "Deep Tissue" certification, even though there is no consensus about what that means, except that spas can often charge more money for the same time slot and therapists are expected to press harder. This revised edition of *Deep Tissue Massage* attempts to provide a more refined explanation of how to make deep tissue and myofascial release skills the foundation of one's practice, regardless of the specialization.

When I began massage in the 1980s, therapists would debate the appropriateness of the terms "massage therapist" or "bodyworker" as the two primary distinctions to define their practices. Now, the prospective student is confronted with a bewildering array of choices for career direction, as each school or teacher seems to offer a proprietary title for what they teach. This is not to say that there isn't extremely important progress in knowledge being offered to both new students and established therapists, but rather that the basic tenets of effective touch remain the same; that is, some of the new nomenclature is simply salesmanship. "A rose by any other name would smell as sweet." I hear from therapists who feel intimidated by the pressure to specialize in a particular niche of bodywork when they would prefer to have the benefits of an eclectic set of tools and the fun of working with a diverse client base.

I even sense a form of elitism as specialists appear to condescend to "regular" massage therapists. Just as in conventional medicine, general practitioners should continue to be esteemed for the broad range of knowledge and skills that can help a large segment of the population. Refined and effective deep tissue massage skills may not sound particularly fancy, but may be the most satisfactory answer to having a diverse and rewarding practice. That is what this book has to offer.

Practitioners working with the techniques and approaches given here will also have the confidence to serve members of the public who are equally confused by all the options. Should a person with a sore shoulder seek ortho-bionomy, soft tissue mobilization, neuromuscular therapy, orthopedic massage (and if so, which brand?), structural integration, myofascial release, or a list of increasingly specialized massage "secrets," each one infinitely superior to last year's favorite? Such techniques as "anchor and stretch" or "pin and stretch," while satisfactory for sports massage for many decades, just seem too pedestrian when fancier names have sprung up for essentially the same procedure. With all this specialization and semantical upgrades of terminology, let us hope that the term "deep tissue massage" will not someday be as meaningless as walking into a Starbucks and asking for a simple cup of coffee.

One increasingly common question in terminology does need some clarification: since the first publication of this book, the term *myofascial release* has become very popular and is sought by the general population as a treatment. Myofascial release skills are taught very differently by different teachers, but

I consider them to be a major component of deep tissue massage. Basically, any technique that releases fascial holding patterns could be called myofascial release. The important distinction between this term and more general massage is that the practitioner usually works more slowly and actually grabs and stretches short fascia rather than sliding over it. If you grasp the principles in this book and the accompanying video set, then you can with good conscience say that you practice deep tissue work, and that myofascial release is one of the numerous components of your deep tissue skill.

When my publisher asked me to consider a revised edition, I was both excited and intimidated by the flood of potential changes. I began a list of new or expanded material to include and added to it daily until I realized that I was creating the *War and Peace* of massage books. With time, however, I realized that although this book emphasizes the *basics* of effective touch, it also offers plenty of specific techniques and structural theory. I am for the most part content with the goals I set out to accomplish five years ago: making deep tissue massage and myofascial release available to a wide range of bodyworkers, rather than attempting to make an intimidating and very specific recipe that some therapists might feel conflicts with their existing practice.

I would not feel this contentment if not for the wonderful array of other detailed and specialized books available to therapists who want to expand their skills. At the risk of leaving out any number of great writers and educators, I would like to specifically mention the incredibly informative work of Erik Dalton, Whitney Lowe, Michael Stanborough, Paul St. Johns, Stuart Taws, and Ben Benjamins, as well as the innovative understanding of anatomy given to all of us by Drew Biel with his *Trail Guide to the Body*. In addition, Tom Myers, with his *Anatomy Trains,* has made the field of Structural Integration accessible to a wide range of therapists. Although Tom's work may be practiced in a strictly structural setting, its brilliance lies in the fact that his clarification of fascial strains on the human structure can be applied to any form of bodywork, including relaxation-based massage. These great educators make it easy for me to stick to what I do best—demystifying deep tissue massage, cultivating effective touch, and helping therapists to expand their present skills and to more effectively (and without injury) express their own individuality and expertise within the field.

This is not to say that I consider the material in this book to be remedial, simplistic, or fodder for a *Deep Tissue Massage for Dummies*. Like most authors, I receive and am very thankful for the communication and compliments that come from satisfied readers. It is gratifying that a wide range of bodyworkers, from beginning students to long-practicing physical therapists and chiropractors, feel that the information in the first edition has benefited them by transforming their work and making them better practitioners. My greatest satisfaction comes not from demonstrating specific strokes or routines, but from the broad paradigm shifts that some therapists report when they grasp how effective and fun the work can be. Just this week I have received three letters expressing how happy these practitioners are with how they are becoming more effective with deep work and developing a problem-solving mentality.

> *"My practice was instantly transformed [by this book], and what I learned there continues to grow."*

> *"[Deep Tissue Massage] has really changed the way I go about my work. It's been absolutely fantastic. This is how I want to practice massage. I've been uncurling bent shoulders, rolling some people onto their sides, fishing for first ribs, and hitting the scalenes. People love the slow melt, and they've reported real differences in the way they feel in their bodies."*

> *"As soon as I begin working with most folks they immediately notice that I do things differently ... and it has helped me grow a rather successful practice in what I would consider a short time. ... I have been currently working with 20 to 30 people each week consistently for the last three to four months and I have only officially been practicing in Maine for eleven months."*

These therapists don't mention learning fancy strokes or tricks, but say that they have altered the way they approach massage with different touch and intention. I feel very strongly that most massage therapists sell themselves short in their potential to effect important change in their clients, because they are unaware of how a few simple changes in technique, vision, and attention to goals rather than strokes can transform their work.

Today's practitioners may be wondering if they can afford to focus on the basics of effective touch when they might instead be developing expertise in a specialization. However, there are few if any bodywork panaceas, and having an excellent touch and a broad panoply of skills can often help practitioners bring more benefit to a wider range of clients. As I mention in Chapter Four, "If you give a man a hammer, the whole world becomes a nail." It is important to remember that in specializing, it is necessary to exclude, and that practitioners who want to see lots of clients with various needs may need to have diverse tools to treat the different symptoms. Too much specialization can limit effectiveness and shrink the number of clients a person can help.

As the required continuing education hours mount, and the measure of a therapist's excellence is increasingly measured by the number of diplomas on the wall, I notice an unfortunate polarization as some therapists disdainfully state that they long ago quit performing "relaxation" massage. I also encounter relaxation-based therapists digging in to their corner, saying that they do not deal with complaints their clients may have with pain or injury. Many relaxation-based massage therapists adamantly state that they have no interest in joining the ranks of the medically-inclined "therapeutic" practitioners as they imagine the necessity of wearing a white coat, having an expensive office with receptionist and insurance forms, and performing cold and impersonal protocols on a string of wounded clients.

Such generalizations and polarizations are unfortunate. Scientific studies increasingly point to the central nervous system as an important, if not major, factor in pain. This understanding is bringing about exciting new therapies that are more holistic rather than simply treating an area where it hurts. As beneficial as all the specific training to release adhesions or other factors at the site of pain are, we may return to giving relaxation massage its rightful place as a powerful medicine for returning the central nervous system to a more balanced state by reducing the charge of the sympathetic branch of the autonomic nervous system, therefore affecting pain from within.

There really is no need for a dichotomy between relaxation and therapeutic massage. The reality is that almost anyone coming to your practice will have complaints and will be grateful for any help you can offer them, either with a decrease in pain, improvement in mobility, athletic or recreational performance. Conversely, many clients with complaints would love to have some relaxation and nurture provided rather than only focusing upon problem-solving.

After learning to perform deep tissue work on even a few isolated areas, countless students admit that their hesitancy was based more upon insecurity about how to deal with such issues than a well-defined decision to exclude such work. When pressed to define their hesitancy, many admit that they lack confidence in their knowledge of anatomy. Of course this can be solved quite easily with just a little study. Most all of these practitioners felt that it must be necessary to take extensive and expensive trainings to learn how to work this way and were amazed that with a few simple changes in outlook and the addition of some deep tissue skills, they were able to transform their practices to be more rewarding, fun, and successful.

Like the original *Deep Tissue Massage,* this revised edition is accessible for virtually any therapist who wants to learn to effectively work deeply with tissue and to bring about important change through effective touch and an understanding of the different layers of the body. I strongly recommend that readers consider studying the more detailed books or videos I mention in the Suggested Reading list at the end of this book (or any of the large number of other publications available), but just as strongly feel that the elements of touch that are covered here and in my DVD set are useful on their own and as a prerequisite to the mastery of whatever form of specialization a practitioner might choose. If you do decide to specialize, these skills will greatly benefit your efficacy in whatever direction you pursue, but you may be surprised to find no need to specialize when you grasp the basic principles of deep tissue massage.

So ... if I am basically content with the first edition and with the multitude of other informative books available, why should we be publishing a second edition? Some of the changes in this revised edition are designed to make the information more accessible and easy to use. This book is printed on a brighter, higher-grade paper stock to make reading easier and especially to allow for greater clarity and detail in the photographs and anatomy plates. Many therapists have commented that eclectic and easy-to-understand techniques in *Deep Tissue Massage* remain useful to them after many readings, and that they often pull out this manual as a quick review to brush up on specific issues. This new edition now offers an index for quick, easy reference to specific topics for review before the client arrives.

With the dramatic increase in therapeutic referrals for massage and the need to communicate with the medical profession and sometimes bill insurance, many therapists also admit to confusion and trepidation about how to work with these issues. The expanded "Troubleshooting" section of this new edition deals much more extensively with some of the issues in this area. The end of Chapter Five includes suggestions for various forms, for instance, a professional patient intake and a copy of liens for dealing with insurance companies and litigation. Directions for taking acceptable chart notes are also provided. A Suggested Reading list makes recommendations for further exploration with other books.

Also, since many people have mentioned purchasing the accompanying DVD set, *Deep Tissue Massage and Myofascial Release: A Video Guide to Techniques,* we have added throughout this book a simple system for referencing the corresponding section in the DVD set. This system affords the advantage of actually seeing the work performed and more effectively learning the all-important subjective qualities of speed and depth of touch.

I hope that you enjoy the information given here and find it useful in a never-ending quest to improve your skills. May your bodywork always be a source of inspiration and fulfilment.

Art Riggs
January 2007

Introduction

THE STUDY OF BODYWORK COULD PERHAPS BE COMPARED TO THE STUDY of mathematics in that there is a natural progression of knowledge and skills that is contingent upon prior training. It is impossible to learn calculus without first having studied algebra. In the same way, as excellent as most introductory massage certification programs are, it would be unwise and unsafe to both the student and the client to attempt to teach anything more than just the rudimentary skills of Deep Tissue Massage until basic massage techniques have been mastered. After several months or years in their practice, many therapists find that their knowledge of the human body has grown, their skills are more sophisticated, and that they desire to contact the body more deeply at both a physical and emotional level, and they are now ready to learn to work at deeper levels.

Students often come to class with some trepidation about beginning to work more deeply. This is a healthy reservation, for deep tissue work takes time to master. However, with the modern emphasis on speed, people want to become experts in a few hours or days. They rush off from weekend workshops considering themselves to be experts. A friend of mine calls this, "ignorance with confidence." This book is intended to expand your ways of looking at the body and the ways you work and can best be used as an adjunct to a Deep Tissue Certification Program at a licensed school. *Deep Tissue Massage: A Visual Guide to Techniques* is not a recipe book to be followed blindly, but with proper training the techniques and theories presented here can be molded to your style, your personality, and the needs of your clients so that you may express your own unique creativity while deepening your practice.

Note: The photographs in this manual show the model wearing underclothes and without draping to cover her body. It is hoped that this does not give too clinical an ambiance to the procedures shown. This format was chosen in order to demonstrate variations in body position with greater clarity. Except for the seated and standing techniques, all of the techniques that are shown can be utilized in a conventional massage in a nurturing manner while using a drape to cover the client.

What Is Deep Tissue Massage?

IT MAY BE HELPFUL TO DISPEL some of the misconceptions before defining Deep Tissue Massage. Most important, it is not a rote technique consisting of prescribed strokes or the use of increasingly powerful "artillery" such as knuckles, fists, or elbows. One of my biggest concerns in writing a book about Deep Tissue Massage was the fear that readers would simply try to mimic the strokes that are shown, without an understanding of how to work deeply *with* (not *on*) tissue. Deep tissue work is not painful and can be very nurturing. Deep work is not satisfying your clients' misconceptions about painful work being more effective—the fallacy of "no pain, no gain."

◎ A deep massage is not a "hard" massage, which is simply the result of exerting more effort; it does not require exceptional strength or size.

Deep Tissue Massage does not require significantly more effort than lighter massage, and is beneficial for most clients. Many students have expressed the fear that deep work will be exhausting or will exacerbate existing overuse injuries that they already experience from doing more superficial massage. They fear that they will have to let go of their present massage practice and recruit an entirely new clientele—that only athletes, laborers, or masochists want deep work. These fears are quickly dispelled as they learn that the principles can immediately be incorporated into their present massage practice. Having the techniques in the repertoire will only expand the potential for attracting clients and enable them to do more profound work with their present clients while exerting less effort. Their work becomes easier and more effective as they learn the new skills of working deeply with proper body mechanics. The slower pace, the focus required to contact clients in a new way, and the fun of problem solving should leave both therapists and clients refreshed and invigorated.

⊚ A massage should never consist entirely of deep work. This would be overwhelming to the client and exhausting to both client and therapist. Deep tissue techniques are intended to be used when the need arises, perhaps several times during a massage. It is as if you are driving on a country road and must slow down and downshift to a more powerful gear when encountering hills or sharp curves.

But what is Deep Tissue Massage? A simple definition might be: *the understanding of the layers of the body, and the ability to work with tissue in these layers to relax, lengthen, and release holding patterns in the most effective and energy efficient way possible.* There is no sharp demarcation between a "regular" massage and deep tissue work. Although the specific skills and tools of Deep Tissue Massage may be somewhat quantifiable by qualities such as depth of pressure, speed of strokes, or use of elbows and knuckles, its practice may vary, depending on therapist, setting, and client. Deep Tissue Massage may have a very different definition in a spa from the understanding of it in a chiropractor's office. Some therapists may continue giving relatively light massage while using their elbows and forearms to work more efficiently. Others may occasionally slow down to use deep tissue methods when the need to effectively soften tissues arises.

In Deep Tissue Massage there is less emphasis on pleasure as the primary goal and more emphasis on altering structure and muscle restrictions. This is not to say that the work is not pleasurable. Most clients, once they are accustomed to the benefits of deep tissue work, prefer the increased degree of relaxation, the alleviation of pain, and the longer lasting benefits. This will result in a more successful practice for you.

⊚ The techniques and different emphasis of these deep tissue methods may offer a profound reorientation in the way you work. You may find that the emphasis upon patiently lengthening tissue will empower you to achieve goals with your clients that were inconceivable before.

The alleviation of pain, bringing about better posture, more flexibility, and fluid movement—these are all potential goals that are possible to achieve with deep tissue skills. Whatever the emphasis, it is hoped that the techniques learned in this manual will be useful to a wide range of therapists as they tailor this knowledge to their own individual definition of massage.

Why Study Deep Tissue Massage?

WHY SHOULD YOU TAKE THE TROUBLE to increase your deep tissue skills? Check out the requirements for employment in most spas and medical settings such as chiropractors' offices or physical therapy clinics. Most of these now require a deep tissue certificate. Massage is no longer looked at as an indulgence to be appreciated by a few people who have excess time or money. Now that the medical community is finally recognizing the benefit of massage as an effective treatment for a whole range of complaints, deep tissue skills are becoming a required prerequisite even to apply for a job. Insurance companies even distinguish between generic massage and "Myofascial Release" or "Soft Tissue Mobilization" (insurance-speak for Deep Tissue Massage) by paying for these services at a higher rate. As private clients become more sophisticated, they too are requiring these skills in your private practice.

In the years that I have taught Deep Tissue Massage, therapists have listed many reasons for taking the course. A large number come because they are injured—they have worked too hard; they have worked too fast; they have used improper posture and biomechanics. They have tried to force and control their clients' tissue with agendas that are in conflict with the realities of human physiology. They may have given their clients' needs preference over their own. Most often, as their knowledge of the human body grows and their skills become more sophisticated, they realize how much more there is to know about bodywork and want to be more effective and better at what they do. To promote this increase in knowledge and skill is the purpose of this book.

◎ Note on DVD referencing: As an aid to readers who are using this book in conjunction with the DVD set, references to the DVDs are provided. The reference on page 6, for example, looks like this: (DVD 1, 20:13 through 52:09). This system identifies the number of the DVD, followed by the elapsed time on the DVD where the given section starts. Scroll forward to the appropriate section using your DVD player's time-counter or find the section by title in the menu at the beginning of each DVD. The table of contents booklet that accompanies the DVD set also contains a complete list of section titles and start times.

Safety First: Caveats

I AM ALWAYS GLAD TO SEE STUDENTS ERRING TOWARDS THE SIDE OF CAUTION in the yin/yang of safety versus overly aggressive treatment. The best advice is never to perform any stroke or procedure unless you know that it is totally safe and feel confident about what you are doing. However, just as the Chinese character for danger also means *opportunity,* zones where Deep Tissue Massage could adversely impact nerves or circulation are also areas where massage can free adhesions or impingements and provide significant improvement. Indiscriminate erring too much on the side of caution may be performing a well-meaning disservice to your clients, which can be simply resolved by an educated confidence in your knowledge of potential danger areas.

In beginning massage classes it is impossible to teach how to work carefully around certain structures until a certain level of expertise has been gained. The warnings not to work in the anterior neck, the abdomen and inguinal triangle, and around certain arteries, veins, and superficial nerves are well advised for a beginning student. However, there is a large difference between not working at all or only superficially in an area and learning in more advanced classes how to work safely in the same area.

◎ It is important to distinguish between a mindful, cautious stroke or maneuver and a tentative and unconfident style of massage.

For years, I have observed the trepidation of new students of Deep Tissue Massage as they explore the boundaries of their confidence and safety. It is reassuring to see this concern for the well being of their clients. However, I have come to the conclusion that much of this apparent caution is actually apprehension due to a lack of knowledge about the anatomical structures that require wariness. Unless you know which structures to beware of or work carefully around, the body may become a nebulous minefield of fearful hesitation.

⊚ Imagine walking through your own living room in total darkness. Knowing where your couch, coffee table, TV, lamps, and other furniture are located would enable you to proceed with cautious confidence to navigate through the room. Now imagine walking through an unfamiliar equally dark room filled with furniture. Your attempts at crossing the room would probably be tentative and fearful. Performing a Deep Tissue Massage without an awareness of the potential anatomical danger areas might be compared to walking through that dark, unfamiliar room.

Caveats (DVD 1, 20:13 through 52:09)

It is important to distinguish between the terms *caveat* and *contraindication*. Caveat implies a caution instead of a prohibition of work (contraindication). An awareness of how to work with the following general anatomical structures will add confidence and efficacy to your work.

Arteries and Veins. The major concern in working with blood vessels is the danger of dislodging atherosclerotic plaque or clots, which can travel through the blood stream to cause strokes. The primary area for concern is the cervical area, but any damaged vein can lodge deposits that can travel through large veins to the heart to be pumped through increasingly smaller arteries until they obstruct blood flow. However, this does not mean that you should never work near large veins or arteries. Though many classes automatically tell students never to work in areas where a pulse can be felt, this seems overly cautious, except when working with older or seriously ill clients. Strong pulses can emanate from the axillary, femoral, and carotid arteries and the descending aorta and be felt several inches away from the actual vessel so that feeling a diffuse pulse is not cause for alarm.

When working in an area where you feel a pulse, you should be aware from your studies of precisely where the artery is located. As you work, slowly move closer to the pulse until you can palpate a more clearly pronounced pulse in order to more precisely locate the artery and then move slightly farther away from that pulse so that you will know that you are not directly working on the artery.

Knowing your anatomy can also help in that absence of a pulse can be cause for alarm in major arterial flow areas such as the descending aorta or the carotid area. This could signal an obstruction or even an aneurysm. Although rare, an aneurysm is a swelling of an artery where the wall has broken down. Any work on this condition could cause rupture of the artery and be life threatening. Practice palpating arterial flow with healthy young clients or fellow massage therapists so that you can know what normal pulses feel like and where they are located.

It is always safest to avoid varicose veins, but many therapists completely neglect the tissue beneath these veins. It is very easy to approach tissue deep to varicose veins from an inch or two on either side of the varicosity to provide relief to leg muscles. Be aware that many clients will be overly cautious and fearful of receiving work near varicose veins. It is important to ask if they would like massage to the area and to explain that you will not disturb the veins.

Nerves. Learn where major nerves travel and when working be alert for signs of impingement such as numbness or tingling. Great benefit can be derived from working areas such as the thoracic outlet where nerves are restricted. Simply explain to your client that you are working near a nerve to release restrictions in that area. Instruct clients to inform you immediately if any numbness or tingling occurs, and discontinue work in that specific area. Often, working an inch away from the specific spot where nerve sensations occur will not be problematic. Be sure to use oblique strokes and to work slowly.

Joints. Many of the strokes in this book demonstrate movement of limbs to stretch muscles. Two areas for caution should be mentioned. If a client has had a hip replacement, especially within the last year, slow, gentle movements are appropriate, but do not attempt to move the joint through full range of motion for a normal hip. Be particularly cautious of flexing the hip while internally rotating the femur and of extending the hip joint while externally rotating the femur. **(DVD 1, 34:24 Hip Replacement Safety Restrictions)**

Unstable shoulder joints are more common. Always move slowly when moving this joint. Most clients will inform you if they have shoulders that are prone to dislocation. In this case, it is safest not to abduct the arm beyond a line perpendicular to the body and to be particularly careful of external rotation of the humerus when the arm is abducted away from the body.

The following photographs list many of the anatomical structures that require a certain degree of care when performing massage. The list is by no means all-inclusive, but does mention some areas that are often not mentioned in beginning massage classes. The best way to learn to work around these areas is to take a hands-on class with an experienced instructor. If you take the time to study these areas and take classes that give protocols for these areas and for medical conditions that require extra care, you will be able to work with confidence.

Areas for Caution

1. **Thoracic Outlet.** This is an area between the anterior and medial scalenes rather than a specific anatomical structure. The radial, ulnar, and median nerves, large circulatory vessels, including the common carotid artery, and jugular veins all traverse this area. Deep Tissue Massage is extremely effective in treating muscular and fascial tightness, which can depress the clavicles against the first rib in this area, and in softening and lengthening the scalene and sternocleidomastoid muscles. Working with muscles that lie in this area is also crucial to provide balance between the front and back of the neck.

2. **Common Carotid Artery.** A strong pulse will alert you to the presence of this artery. Do not press directly on the artery, but learn to work carefully on tissue that is adjacent to it. Particular care is needed with older or unhealthy clients because of the danger of clots or plaque deposits, which could be dislodged with massage.

3. **Carotid Sinus.** This is a particular section of the carotid artery that is a baroceptor; it is sensitive to and regulates blood pressure. Direct pressure on this structure can initiate a precipitous drop in blood pressure.

4. **Brachial Plexus.** This plexus of nerves lies directly above the clavicle, but can be impinged by fascial restrictions more than an inch away. Working with the lower origins of the scalenes can elicit nerve sensations in this plexus. Always inform your client to alert you if any numbness or tingling is felt in the arm when working in this area. If you are working slowly and carefully, this is not dangerous; all that is necessary is to move slightly farther away or work in a slightly different oblique angle after symptoms have subsided.

5. **Parotid Salivary Gland.** The seventh (facial) nerve travels through this gland.

6. **Submandibular Salivary Gland.** This gland lies beneath and along the inferior line of the mandible. Lymph nodes also lie beneath the submandibular salivary gland.

7. **Axillia.** This area contains lymph nodes and a neurovascular bundle. Unless there are specific therapeutic reasons to be working in this area, it is best to avoid it.

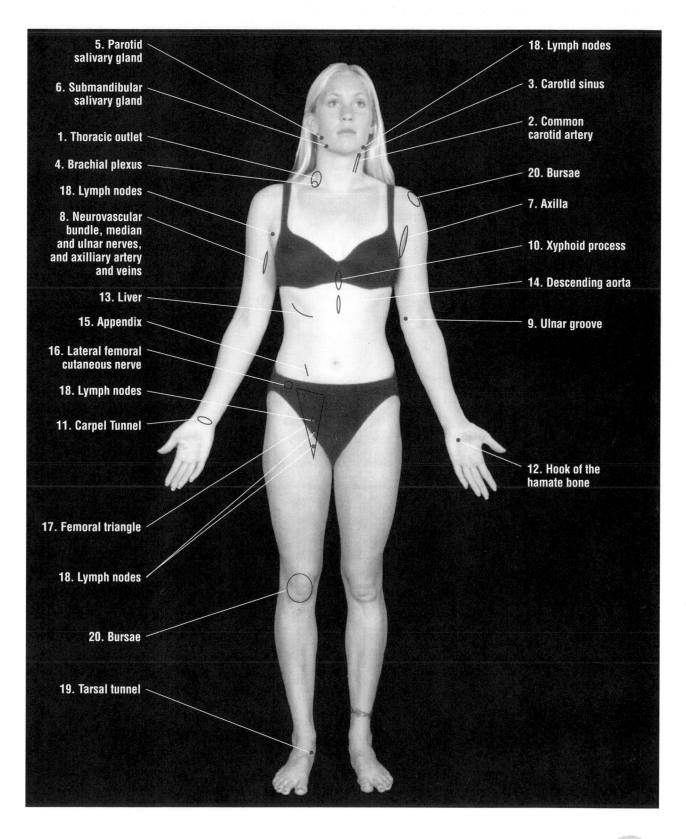

5. Parotid salivary gland

6. Submandibular salivary gland

1. Thoracic outlet

4. Brachial plexus

18. Lymph nodes

8. Neurovascular bundle, median and ulnar nerves, and axilliary artery and veins

13. Liver

15. Appendix

16. Lateral femoral cutaneous nerve

18. Lymph nodes

11. Carpel Tunnel

17. Femoral triangle

18. Lymph nodes

20. Bursae

19. Tarsal tunnel

18. Lymph nodes

3. Carotid sinus

2. Common carotid artery

20. Bursae

7. Axilla

10. Xyphoid process

14. Descending aorta

9. Ulnar groove

12. Hook of the hamate bone

8. **Neurovascular Bundle, Median and Ulnar Nerves, and Axilliary Artery and Veins.** These structures lie between the biceps and triceps approximately half way down the humerus.

9. **Ulnar Groove.** The ulnar nerve lies close to the bony surface of the elbow.

10. **Xyphoid Process.** Avoid direct pressure on this bone; there is very little reason to justify working directly on it.

11. **Carpal Tunnel.** The median nerve travels though the carpal tunnel. Be careful not to compress this area, but spreading tissue on either side can open the channel to provide less compression in the area.

12. **Hook of the Hamate Bone.** This bony protrusion in the palm of the hand is easily palpated. The ulnar nerve can be compressed with direct pressure on the hamate bone, so avoid such pressure.

13. **Liver.** Be cautious of applying deep pressure directly beneath the costal arch when working with the diaphragm in this area.

14. **Descending Aorta.** Refer to broad circulatory discussion earlier in this section.

15. **Appendix.** There would be no reason to attempt to work directly on the appendix. However, if general abdominal work elicits sharp painful sensations in this area, it could indicate an inflamed appendix, particularly if the client complains of malaise or fever.

16. **Lateral Femoral Cutaneous Nerve.** This nerve passes directly under the inguinal ligament. This is not a common area to be accessing in a massage, but may be encountered when working with the psoas, iliacus, or the origin of muscles at the anterior superior iliac spine.

17. **Femoral Triangle.** The femoral artery and veins, femoral nerve, and lymph nodes and vessels descend through this area.

18. **Lymph Nodes.** You will not want to actually massage any lymph nodes, but should be able to determine if any nodes are swollen or too hard. In this case, it is best to avoid the area.

19. **Tarsal Tunnel.** The posterior tibial nerve, artery, and vein travel below the medial malleolus.

20. **Bursae.** Anywhere a tendon crosses a joint, there is a possibility that a bursa will be cushioning the tendon from rubbing against bone. Major areas for bursae are the shoulder, hip, knee, and elbow. Bursae do not respond well to massage, although working around them may provide relief to traumatized joints. Often clients will inform you that they have bursitis of a particular joint. It is a good idea to determine if this is actually an educated diagnosis from a medical professional or a guess from someone less

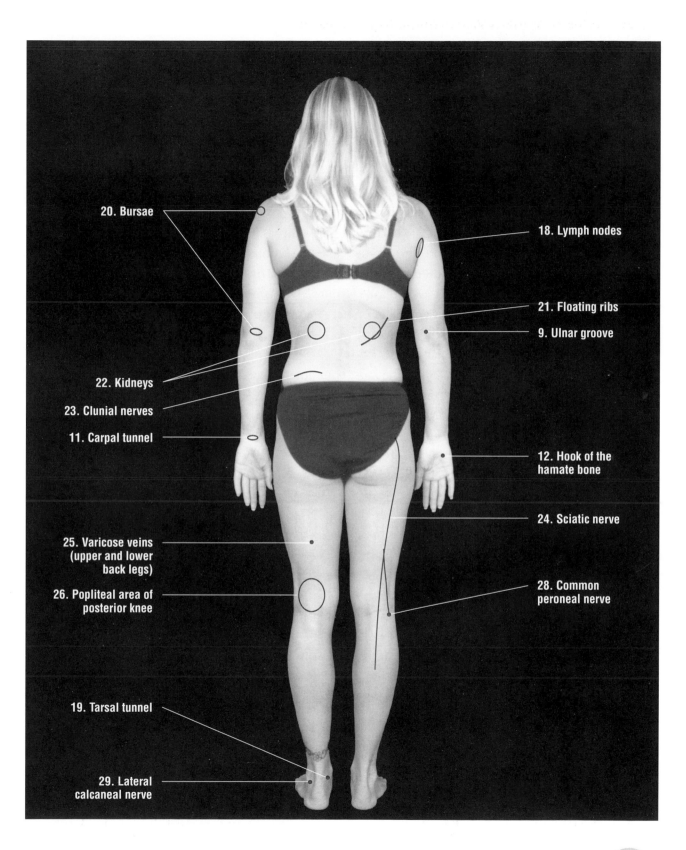

20. Bursae

18. Lymph nodes

21. Floating ribs

9. Ulnar groove

22. Kidneys

23. Clunial nerves

11. Carpal tunnel

12. Hook of the hamate bone

25. Varicose veins (upper and lower back legs)

24. Sciatic nerve

26. Popliteal area of posterior knee

28. Common peroneal nerve

19. Tarsal tunnel

29. Lateral calcaneal nerve

qualified. Bursitis and tendonitis are often confused and their treatments are very different. Sensitive tendons often respond well to cross-fiber friction massage and ice, while bursitis can be inflamed by work and responds well to heat.

21. **Floating Ribs.** These bottom ribs are not attached to the costal cartilage or the sternum and are more mobile and delicate. Do not apply broad pressure here because of the mobility of the floating ribs and the presence of the kidneys below them.

22. **Kidneys.** The floating ribs lie directly over the kidneys. Avoid excessive direct pressure on the ribs; work obliquely in this area.

23. **Clunial Nerves.** Although the crest of the ilium is an important area to address, use oblique strokes. This is not a common area for warning, but if clients comment on nerve sensations in the buttocks when you are working on the iliac crest, work slightly away from the specific area that elicits these sensations.

24. **Sciatic Nerve.** The most common area compression of this nerve could occur during massage is at the piriformis muscle and between the ischial tuberosity and the trochanter. Be sure to use oblique strokes in the entire gluteal area so that nerves are not compressed against the pelvis.

25. **Varicose Veins.** Refer to broad circulatory discussion earlier in this section.

26. **Popliteal Area of Posterior Knee.** Slow and careful work can be very productive in the posterior knee area to relax the hamstring and gastrocnemius tendons and the popliteus and plantaris muscles. The popliteal and tibial nerves and the popliteal artery and vein also travel posterior to the synovial capsule of the knee.

27. **Squamous Portion of the Temporal Bone and the Greater Wing of the Sphenoid Bone.** These bones of the skull are very thin in this area. The sphenoid is relatively mobile for a cranial bone and can be displaced by pressure. Use only the most gentle, oblique pressure in this area.

28. **Common Peroneal Nerve.** This nerve is most vulnerable directly behind the fibular head.

29. **Lateral Calcaneal Nerve.**

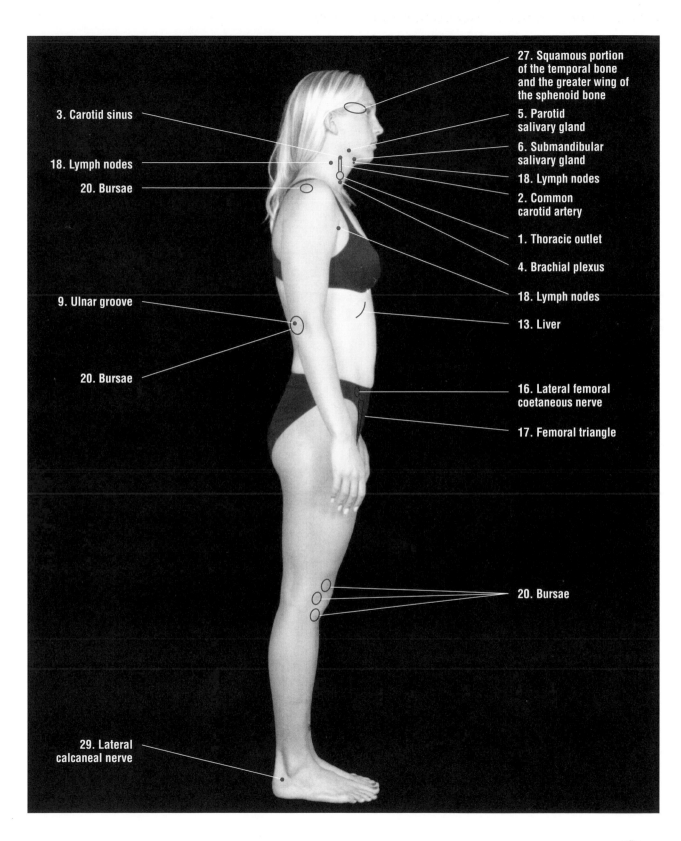

3. Carotid sinus

18. Lymph nodes

20. Bursae

9. Ulnar groove

20. Bursae

29. Lateral
calcaneal nerve

27. Squamous portion
of the temporal bone
and the greater wing of
the sphenoid bone

5. Parotid
salivary gland

6. Submandibular
salivary gland

18. Lymph nodes

2. Common
carotid artery

1. Thoracic outlet

4. Brachial plexus

18. Lymph nodes

13. Liver

16. Lateral femoral
coetaneous nerve

17. Femoral triangle

20. Bursae

Chapter One

General Theories

THE SPECIFIC DEEP TISSUE TECHNIQUES THAT ARE DEMONSTRATED IN this book are based upon broad principles of massage, and must be taught in that context. In reality, the line between relaxation oriented massage and deep tissue work is not a sharp one: even a gentle massage can be made more beneficial by including deep work, and a good Deep Tissue Massage should include considerable time spent on relaxing and nurturing strokes. Deep Tissue Massage is not simply the use of "heavy artillery" such as knuckles, fists, and elbows. Tools can become weapons in the wrong hands, and as tempting as it might be dive in with our elbows, it is necessary to spend some time talking about how to work with tissue safely and effectively. The following principles will clarify the theories upon which the specific techniques demonstrated in later chapters are based. **(DVD 1, 0:16 Fundamentals of DTM and MR)**

Principles of Deep Tissue Massage

Never strain: Working deep is different from working hard. If you strain or notice that you are shaking from attempting to work too hard, either work less hard, work more slowly, or switch to a different "tool" such as an elbow or forearm. It is very difficult to dissipate stress in a client's body if you are imposing stress from working beyond your capacity.

Use little oil. Oil or lotion is, of course, necessary to prevent skin friction; however, most students use much more than is necessary. If you have ever attempted to turn a doorknob with oily hands, you know how much effort you need to accomplish this simple task. When working deeply, it is crucial to your well-being that you not strain or "effort." Too much lubricant dissipates your energy at the layer of the skin rather than at the depth where you are trying to work, requiring you to waste your energy. Lotions are usually less slippery than oils and allow you to more easily grab tissue without applying too much pressure.

Work slowly. Working deeply requires a reciprocal relationship between the speed of the stroke and the depth of work. The more deeply you work or the greater the resistance of the muscles to relaxing, the more slowly you must work. When people associate pain with deep work, it is usually the speed of work rather than the depth or amount of pressure that is responsible.

Use oblique pressure. Never push directly towards the bone. One should rarely work at an angle greater than forty-five degrees. Nerves and blood vessels have the ability to stretch or move from side to side, but may be injured if impinged against bone. This is particularly important in the gluteal area where the sciatic nerve is easily impinged against the pelvis. Oblique pressure also allows you to stretch tissue rather than merely compressing it.

Work tendinous insertion of muscles in addition to working the belly of muscles. Often the stress of overworked or chronically short and inflexible muscles manifests itself at the attachment of the tendon to the bone. Softening the tendon and stimulating the stretch receptors (Golgi tendon organs) is important to effect a relaxation of the muscles. This is particularly important with long muscles such as the hamstrings. Working the insertion may relax the muscle enough that less time will be needed with meticulous work on the belly of the muscle.

Have a clear intention of what you want to accomplish. Evaluate each client visually, by palpation, and by questioning them to determine the major areas where tension is held. Too many massage therapists simply begin working the same way with all clients and massage "by the numbers." This translates to an emphasis on style rather than substance. Most of us have experienced a massage where the strokes are performed with great flourish and flare only to have perfunctory attention paid to areas that are crying out for extra attention. Your goals should dictate your techniques.

Direct attention to the layer of the body at which you want to work and continue at that layer. The nervous system is sensitive to the different depths of stimulation it receives. Moving quickly from one layer to another can have the effect of relaxing individual muscles while at the same time overstimulating the nervous system. Slowly sink to the layer where you intend to work; continue working at the layer, and then slowly withdraw. Having a firm basis of anatomical knowledge, including knowledge of muscle origins and insertions, will aid in establishing a strategy of work and understanding mobility restrictions and rotational patterns.

Let the body react and stabilize before moving on. Beginning classes sometimes over-emphasize the importance of taking care not to upset the body's energy field by instructing students to not break contact with the body during a massage. However, constant stimulation may have the effect of preventing the client from integrating and stabilizing. Profound changes in the form of a deep sigh, sweating, the relaxation of a chronically short muscle, and changes of skin color are signs of autonomic nervous system activity. If you notice these changes, it is often a good idea to stop actively working and even break contact with the client for a short time to let the relaxation solidify and be remembered either consciously or subconsciously.

In most cases, put muscles into a stretched position to effect a release. The vast majority of problems we encounter are a result of short, contracted muscles. Therapists are often hesitant to move limbs or reposition the client for fear of disturbing the state of relaxation. However, if a tight muscle is placed in an easy stretch near its end range, when the muscle relaxes, it will lengthen. For all practical purposes this educates the muscle stretch receptors to reestablish a new definition of what its resting length is. Many of the positions shown in this book are designed to place muscles into stretched positions while you are working.

For example, visualize the length of the biceps muscles with the arm flexed at approximately a forty-five degree angle as it might rest in a massage if your client is in the supine position. You could be successful in softening the biceps, but your client would probably stand up with his arm bent at the same angle as when he arrived. However, extending the elbow to stretch the biceps while you were working would actually lengthen the muscle. But take care to not overstretch muscles. If stretched too much, they will be difficult to access deeply or will contract against the stretch.

Use proper body mechanics. Most injuries to therapists come from straining in their work. This can come from working too fast or from improper body mechanics. The energy for your work should not come from contraction of your own muscles. Either use gravity and your own weight directed from above, or have the force come from your feet as you push from the ground. Throughout this book, suggestions will be offered to improve body mechanics.

Don't use thumbs for any deep work. The thumbs are too important a tool in general massage to be exhausted or injured performing deep work. Ninety percent of the deep work that is usually performed by the thumbs can be accomplished by knuckles, fists, or even elbows. Practice with these tools, and they will feel as comfortable and effective as your thumbs.

Reading the Body

THE BEST THERAPISTS SEEM TO KNOW AUTOMATICALLY where tension is held in a client's body. This skill is not something they are born with; it evolves from practice. It can come from visual, tactile, verbal, and intuitive cues. Tension and holding patterns a client reveals while standing or walking may not manifest themselves when the client is lying on the table, so utilize the moments you have with the client before she is resting on the table. When a client comes into the room, immediately attempt to determine two or three areas that might be areas of holding. Does one hip swing freely while the other is immobile? Does one arm hang with ease while the elbow of the other arm is rigid and transmits tension to the shoulder? Is the mid-back pain a response to tightness in the chest? Corroborate these impressions throughout the massage. This will cultivate your visual awareness. (For a more detailed explanation of bodyreading evaluation of strain patterns, see Chapter Six.)

A massage should be a blending of your evaluation (intake) and manipulation (output). In reality, evaluative palpation for tension is therapeutic and is an effective use of time in relaxing the client. When the client is on the table, take a few moments to assess the whole body rather than just beginning to work on one isolated spot. Palpate major muscle groups to feel for tightness or spasm. Gently rock the body and notice any rotational or holding patterns. Distract joints by pulling or shaking arms and legs. In addition to softening muscles, the goal of a massage should be to give a feeling of connection between various body segments, and making contact with the body as a whole can provide this. How fluid is the connection between the hips and low back? The ankle and the leg? The leg and the pelvis? The occiput and the cervicals? Do restrictions seem to be a result of immobile joints (i.e. tight ligaments or calcification) or a result of soft tissue restrictions? Which of these areas do you want to concentrate on?

If you are working in a one-hour format, spending a lot of time on palpation and bodyreading may be difficult. However, even a minute or two of evaluation before the active massage begins will give you important cues for planning a strategy and will quickly relax the client and integrate the body. Such evaluation should continue throughout the massage—let it be a constant interplay of work and reading the messages of the body.

Constant "listening" to the messages of the client not only allows for a better massage; it frees the therapist from the boredom of mindless repetition of the same routine for every client. Students often report that with this approach burnout is eliminated and massage becomes fun again.

Refining Your Touch

THERE ARE MANY CAUSES OF INJURIES TO THERAPISTS; almost all of them are a result of working too hard. Some students fear doing deep tissue work because they are already exhausted from more shallow work and already have injuries. However, proper use of these techniques should enable anyone to work with more ease and safety, and also make the work more effective and enjoyable. It is important to make a distinction between *deep* and *hard*. Deep work is just that—deep. It does not have to be painful or exhausting to either the client or therapist. It is crucial to learn to sink into the tissue slowly, moving only as fast as the client allows. Not all muscles are ready to relax. Even with perfect technique and tactile sensitivity, it can be exhausting if the therapist attempts to force a release upon the client who is not ready to relax. Work slowly and *let,* not *make* relaxation happen.

The photographs in this manual are only suggestions of postures that will enable you to more effectively express your touch in order to contact your clients at a deeper level. They are not a substitute for diligent study, practice, and experimentation to refine your sensitivity and touch. It is highly recommended that you learn and practice techniques in this book with supervision. More than one technique can be used to achieve the same goal; do not feel limited to imitating exactly what is shown.

ⓞ Some of the techniques shown in this manual will not be appropriate for some therapists and some will not be appropriate for some clients. When you are familiar with the techniques that work best for you, there should be an ease and flow to your work that will feel effortless. These techniques are only the beginning—feel free to experiment and express yourself. The joy of our work is the escape from rigidity in our techniques in order to express our creativity and intuition in a constant interplay with the client.

Quality of Touch

ⓞ Imagine that you are receiving a massage from a total stranger. . . . How long does it take for you to determine the quality of the massage you are about to receive? Most people respond that they know within the first two or three minutes of the massage, simply by the initial quality of touch that the therapist demonstrates.

A quality massage is not just fancy strokes or sophisticated techniques. I have received wonderful work from relatively inexperienced massage therapists who have a good touch. I have also counted the minutes until the massage is finished when receiving work from graduates of 1000-hour trainings who have a huge repertoire of strokes and have been practicing for many years, but have not cultivated their touch.

A massage, whether a gentle energetic experience or an extremely deep session, is a dance between you and your client. Anyone who has danced, either as a leader or as a follower, knows the joy of having a partner who is present at all times and reacts to the smallest cue. As therapists we are in the role of leading, but it is essential to constantly be reading the responses of our clients. Some people need more direction or are more comfortable with a different tempo. Many therapists attempt to dance the same dance with every client. However, your strategy will be dictated by many factors—your emotional connection and the reciprocal trust between you and your client, the quality of tissue and holding patterns (primarily at a localized tissue level or more a result of neurological or emotional holding patterns), areas of pain or fear in your client, and countless other subtle factors.

How to Cultivate Your Touch

Acting on the following suggestions can improve your skills and help you cultivate your touch.

Receive Work from Accomplished Bodyworkers

It is surprising how often students admit that they rarely receive bodywork except for occasional trades with fellow students. They become mired in a vicious circle of not having enough clients, worrying about the expense of getting work from experts, and never learning the sensations of cultivated touch. They fail to improve the quality of their work and as a result their practices fail to grow.

Paying for work from experienced experts always pays off. You receive excellent work on your own body, and, just as important, you always learn skills to apply to your own practice. Ask the therapist to explain what she is doing during the massage. I am always amazed at how enthusiastic I am after receiving work. Not only do I learn new ways of working, but my confidence in my own work grows as I realize similarities in our styles and the benefit we give our clients. Budget your finances to receive work on a regular basis and make that appointment now!

Take Continuing Education Classes

I know therapists who have not taken a class in years. Some of them are hesitant to spend the money or to take the time off from work or play. Others have full practices or only consider classes for their potential to generate more income or fulfill obligations for continuing education or licensing. However, consider that in taking classes you not only learn, but will also receive several hours of good work on your own body from your peers.

Consider taking classes in different disciplines, as very different types of work can expand your skills. The most profound effect upon the deep work I do with Rolfing® came from the subtle skills I learned in two craniosacral classes.

Schedule a Tutorial

If you have a teacher whom you respect, arrange for yourself and a friend to take a few hours of training in a non-classroom environment. Define what you wish to get out of the session. The teacher should not only observe and comment on your work on each other, but also should also be open to receiving your work so that she can comment on your touch.

Ask to give a teacher a massage in exchange for feedback even though it can be intimidating. Make it clear that you are open to constructive criticism and welcome any suggestions on how to improve your work. You should expect the session to be much more than just a free massage for your teacher followed by broad comments on how much she enjoyed the massage. When I receive work from students, I often jump off the table many times during a session to offer suggestions and demonstrations about biomechanics, strategies, and the quality of touch I am experiencing. After the massage we sit down and discuss the strong points of the massage and also potential areas for improvement. Be aware that it is customary to pay the teacher for such services.

Practice Palpation (DVD 1, 9:30)

Work on yourself. Evaluate what your own touch feels like. Experiment with speed of strokes, what it feels like to stretch tissue rather than just sliding over the skin. Palpate deep muscles through superficial muscles. Begin to get a sense of how the neck functions, differentiating rotation, side-bending, flexion, and extension at each separate cervical vertebra. (Chapters Three and Four give information about working with the neck.)

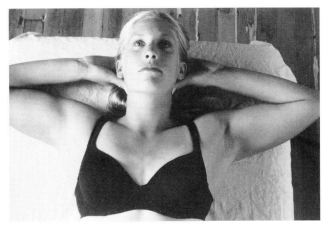

Figure 1-1

Figure 1-1. Self-Palpation of the Cervicals

Lie on your back and place your hands on each side of your cervical vertebrae as shown. Try to locate the transverse processes of your atlas by moving caudally approximately one-half inch below your mastoid process. Proceed down your spine feeling the transverse processes of each vertebra. Feel for tender or sore areas on the transverse processes and in the small intervertebral muscles in order to train your fingers to sense what inflammation feels like. This sensitivity will enable you to find similar areas of pain in your clients. Notice what type of pressure is necessary to cause a softening of tissue.

Train your fingers to be constantly sensing and working with different aspects of both living and non-living things. Try to differentiate the partitions in a tangerine or orange through the skin. See if you can free the skin of a banana from the fruit without bruising it. Notice the difference in tissue quality in different animals such as cats and dogs and try to touch them in different ways, seeing if you can anticipate their responses if you work too hard.

Cultivate a sensitive touch. The following experiment is very popular in classes: Students mention it years after class as one of the most helpful demonstrations they have experienced. Take a box of cornstarch and empty it into a fairly deep bowl so that it will be a few inches deep. Mix in approximately one and one-half cups of water slowly until the texture resembles the texture of shoe polish. Experiment with the mixture, sinking into it with hands and finger, and noticing its reaction to your pressure. If you slide your fingers with pressure across the top, you will notice that it actually *tears,* similar to the potential for microtears to tissue from too fast strokes. Pound the cornstarch with your fist and notice how it responds to your force by becoming hard and resistant. Try to push your fingers as quickly as you can to the bottom and notice how much effort it takes.

Now let your fingers *sink* into the mixture with very little effort and notice how much you can accomplish when your pressure and speed are unforced. Remove your hand quickly from the cornstarch and notice how the entire mixture clings to your fingers. Remember that that the speed that you withdraw from tissue is almost as important as how you sink into tissue. *Take the time to do this demonstration!* I've had physical therapists who have been practicing for years say that this helped their touch more than any single exercise they have ever practiced.

Some Aspects That Define Touch

A Soft Touch

The depth at which you work has little correlation with how *hard* you work. This one aspect has been a constant struggle for me; being relatively strong, I have a natural tendency to simply apply more effort when I encounter resistance. Each year I practice, I find that I accomplish more with less effort.

◎ Our role is to release tension in the body. It is counterproductive to attempt to teach relaxation to our clients by imposing tension with stiff fingers or by muscular straining. Elimination of strain is influenced by many factors such as your own strength and weight, proper biomechanics, the speed of your strokes, the amount of lubrication you use, and most important, awareness of your client's response to your work. If your client is resisting your efforts, applying more force is rarely the solution.

Always be alert for signs of strain in your own body. If your hands become hard and inflexible or you notice shaking when you are working, it is a sure sign that you need to work less hard. It is mentally and physically exhausting and you risk injury to yourself and your client if you attempt to force relaxation.

◎ This ability to work without strain utilizes an unspoken contract between you and your client which I call **surrender.** Both of you must let go of or surrender your will in a compromise based upon trust. Surrender is not a defeat or loss of power. As the therapist, you must let go of any agendas about forcing muscles to relax. You can only facilitate an opening and relaxation by **letting** it happen, not by **making** it happen. It involves letting go of attempting to control the outcome. Without this, the massage can become a power struggle between you and your client. If your clients can sense your compassion and flexibility, they can surrender their resistance to change without a feeling of defeat or of surrendering their power.

The Distinction Between Compressing Tissue and Stretching Tissue

Along with having a soft and nurturing touch, this is the most important quality I attempt to teach in classes. Imagine a tire rolling over soft ground. . . . This is the quality of compression—a useful massage technique, but very different from stretching tissue. With compression, we may improve circulation, soften muscles and affect energy, but often the tissue will retain its length. However, most tissue that we influence is not only *hard*, but is also *short*. To increase your effectiveness it is essential to be able to lengthen short tissue.

(Notice the distinction between the terms *muscle* and the more complex term, *tissue,* which includes fascia, muscles, and tendons.)

Now imagine pulling taffy.... The ability to lengthen tissue is what will separate you from the vast majority of therapists and will increase your effectiveness and ensure the repeat clients necessary for a full practice. Stretching tissue requires an awareness of the depth at which you are working, the use of oblique pressure, an ability to *grab* or *snowplow* tissue, and a knowledge of kinesiology in order to place your client into positions that will stretch muscles. Most of the different techniques demonstrated in this book are designed to lengthen areas of shortness.

Biomechanics (DVD 1, 15:28)

If a bodyworker's body is tense, this tension will be conveyed to the client. Thus, proper use of your own body weight and having your energy come from your *core* rather than from muscular effort is an essential part of remaining healthy and refreshed and providing a touch that is healing. Proper table height is essential for this, and though classes sometimes give universal rules for table height, there are no ideal table heights for everyone. A therapist with low back problems will probably need a relatively high table to keep a more upright posture, while someone with shoulder problems might need a lower table in order to use his own weight rather than muscular effort to provide power.

A therapist's position also needs to vary depending on client position or part of the body being worked on. I see students going to great lengths to measure a table's height or even have a fellow student get off the table to lower it one notch when working on the upper back, only to find that the table is too low to properly work on the feet. Many of the techniques in this book employ the side-lying position. This might mean that you are working at a height that is eight or more inches higher than when your client is lying in prone or supine position. The solution often lies in using another tool such as elbows or fists or moving closer or farther away from the table to utilize a different angle for working.

If you work at an office rather than doing out-call massage, seriously consider purchasing an electric adjustable table. Your clients will understand if you raise your rates a small amount, and the table will be paid for in a few months. You will be amazed at how refreshed you will feel and how much more effective your work will be when your table is always at the right height at the push of a foot pedal.

Proper Working Distance from a Client

Proper working distance from your client is also important to convey a touch that is both relaxed and powerful. Power should come from two basic sources: *gravity* allows for the *weight* of the therapist to be directed from above the client. At an oblique angle, the feet and the legs should provide the force from the ground. Most of the therapist's joints should be extended but not locked. If you work too close to the client with bent arms, force must be supplied by the external muscles rather than from core energy. However, if you work too far away, you will not have the use of your own weight and gravity at your disposal.

Figure 1-2. Ideal Working Distance

In this example, the therapist is far enough away that the wrists, elbows, shoulders, and back are all extended so that no energy is lost at bent joints when pushing with the legs. The therapist is also close enough that he may use his own weight to supply pressure from above.

Figure 1-3. Working Too Close

Here we see that the therapist is too close to the client. Note the flexed right wrist, bent elbows, compressed shoulders, and forward flexion at the waist. If the therapist wanted to use gravity more effectively, he could climb on the table so the arms would be extended or could use another tool such as the forearm.

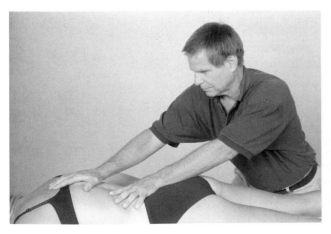

Figure 1-2

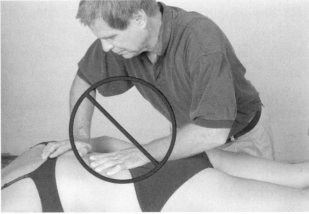

Figure 1-3

Figure 1-4. Ideal Working Distance— Combining Gravity and Horizontal Power

This illustrates a compromise between use of the legs for horizontal power and of the therapist's own body weight for depth. Notice that the limbs are all extended so that no power is lost.

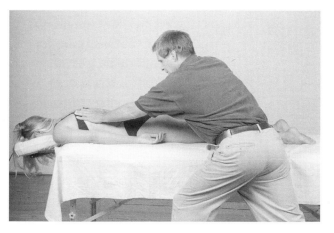

Figure 1-4

◎ It is important to note that in Figure 1-4 the therapist is working unilaterally. Many students attempt to always work both sides of the spine at the same time. Particularly with a short therapist and a tall client, you may only be able to work effectively half way down the back before your use of gravity is lost. There are many other reasons for working on one side of the spine at a time; for instance, rib or spinal rotations may benefit from working up on one side and down on the other. Also, muscular tension is often significantly different from one side of the spine to the other, and more focused work on one side is needed.

Figure 1-5. Too Far Away

The therapist is too far away to use his own body weight to work with anything but superficial pressure. Notice that the forward bend at the waist prevents efficient use of the legs to supply energy, and that any depth of pressure must be supplied by the muscular effort of extending the arms downward rather than using gravity.

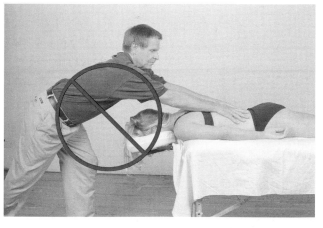

Figure 1-5

The All-Important Melt of Muscle Tissue

One of the key elements to refined touch is the ability to feel subtle responses in your clients' tissue. Some therapists are so intent on their *strokes* that they are unresponsive to the changes taking place in tissue. If you do not sense the softening of muscle, how will you know when your work is finished? Most of us have experienced the frustration of having a therapist mindlessly repeat strokes when a tight area has already relaxed and softened. At the other end

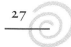

of the continuum, it is equally frustrating to have someone grind away at tissue that is not responding. Often, strokes are performed so quickly that it is impossible to evaluate their effect. However, one of the great rewards of our work is to experience the successful softening as a response to our efforts.

Having the patience to work slowly and wait for the tissue to soften or melt is the key to deep tissue work. The therapist will be unlikely to experience overuse injuries and will have the satisfaction of feeling the changes in their clients' bodies. Clients will not experience pain and will be more integrated with less stress to the nervous system.

To accomplish this melt, it helps to visualize pushing a heavy boat away from a dock. You would not get a running start—you would slowly push. At first, you might not feel any movement, but eventually you would sense the accumulated effort have an effect. As inertia is conquered, less force is required and you can relax your effort and pay more attention to other factors such as direction of movement or *unwinding*. The best way to experience this is to feel it in your own body; find an area of tension and experiment on yourself. When you feel an area release or melt, it is sometimes beneficial to point it out to the client so that they can remember to keep the area relaxed.

A Few Words about Pain

THE SUBJECT OF DISCOMFORT OR PAIN often comes up in classes. Many people who request deep work expect some discomfort, and the line between discomfort and pain is often not a sharp one. It sometimes helps to clarify that line with clients by having them describe what they are feeling. For some people, any intense sensation is described as pain. Having them articulate the sensation will often clarify that what is actually experienced is a feeling of warmth, stretching, or even emotions such as distrust, fear, or anger. Usually, pain is a result of working too quickly and forcing your agenda; slowing down strokes while using the same amount of pressure will often solve the problem. You should not knowingly impose pain on a client. If you feel the client tightening rather than relaxing, you are working too intensely.

For clients with specific problems who are asking for intense work, it is often helpful to have them inform you if the intensity exceeds seven on a scale of ten. Of course, this is a relative term, but having the client involved in the process empowers them and will often help them feel safe enough not to resist the work. Clients should always feel free to verbalize any doubts or fears they may experience with intense work. However, there is a fine line between their freedom to express any reservations and the need that some clients have to attempt to control the massage. One of the joys of receiving work is to be able to relax completely without feeling that feedback is required. Some therapists interrupt the process of relaxing and letting go by too frequently asking for feedback.

◎ Caution: Any shooting pain or numbness is a sign that there is nerve involvement. Immediately stop working deeply on that area.

Direction of Strokes

MOST BEGINNING MASSAGE COURSES TEACH that whenever possible it is a good idea to work in the direction of the blood flow back to the heart. However, this is not an inflexible rule. If you are working slowly enough, there should be no danger of damaging veins if you work in a direction away from the circulatory flow. Joints are often compressed, and having the intention of decompressing or creating space in joints is almost always a worthwhile goal. Rigidly adhering to rules such as *always* working towards the heart may not be the best strategy for tight joint capsules. Sometimes the only way to give a cue to the client to relax holding around a joint that is being overly protected is to work both directions away from the joint. Working in each direction away from the elbow, shoulder, hip, knee, wrist, or ankle is a useful strategy for all of these joints.

Figure 1-6. Decompressing a Joint (DVD 2, 17:46)
Working in a downward direction from the hip joint can give the cue to let the hip and leg drop and create space at a compressed acetabulum.

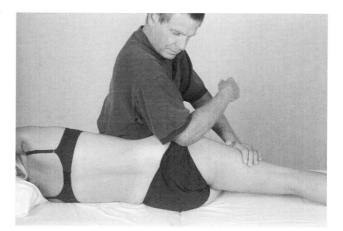

Figure 1-6

Some Basic Stroke Strategies

THERAPISTS SOMETIMES BECOME LOCKED into certain routines of strokes without considering their goals for their clients. This habit is particularly common in spa settings where clients are lined up for fifty-minute massages like planes waiting to land at a busy airport. Such massages are sometimes given names like "cookie cutter" or "by the numbers" massages. Burnout and injury are common as the therapist begins working with as much enthusiasm and imagination as a production line worker. To enjoy your work and stay fresh, it is absolutely essential to look at each client as an individual and to have clear goals and strategies for each massage. Depending upon holding patterns, different parts of an individual may require totally different strokes. The following are some variations.

Lengthening Strokes (DVD 2, 14:26)

These are probably the most commonly used strokes to elongate short muscles. They are often used in light massage, but are also extremely useful for deep tissue work. However, the emphasis upon long flowing strokes can sometimes be carried too far as therapists extend the stroke beyond their range of power. This is an example of emphasizing form over substance or function. Don't be afraid to interrupt a long lengthening stroke part way down the back or leg if you have lost your power or you encounter a particularly tight area.

Also, remember not to use too much lubrication; this will prevent your grabbing and lengthening tissue. Your goal is to stretch and lengthen muscles, not to just compress them by slipping over them.

Anchor and Stretch (DVD 2, 28:47 and 32:04)

Visualize a knot in a rubber band. If you stretch the rubber band, the flexible areas will lengthen, while the knot will remain tight. Tight or fibrosed areas rarely extend the entire length of the muscle, and yet, therapists often give equal attention to the whole muscle. An effective strategy is to anchor at the spot of most tension and to stretch the muscle in either direction from this spot. It is crucial that you not slide on the surface above the holding area. Visualize that you are grabbing the tight area and stretching away from it.

Notice how you can move a limb to stretch a muscle while anchoring on a tight area, as we see in Figures 1-7 and 1-8.

Figure 1-7. Anchor and Stretch (Knee)

Flex the knee to shorten the hamstring. Anchor a particularly tight area and then extend the knee with your other hand to stretch tissue from the point of anchor.

Figure 1-8. Anchor and Stretch (Back)

On any area of the body it is a useful strategy to anchor with one tool and stretch in the opposite direction with the other hand.

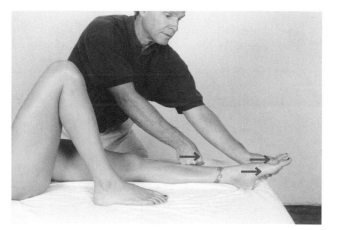

Figure 1-7

Working in the Direction of Stretch

It is effective to extend a muscle's end range by extending a joint while at the same time working the muscle in the direction of lengthening.

Figure 1-9. Working in the Direction of Lengthening

Rather than anchoring at a tight area and stretching away from the spot as in the previous example, extend the ankle from a flexed position and expedite the lengthening of the muscle by applying force in the same direction.

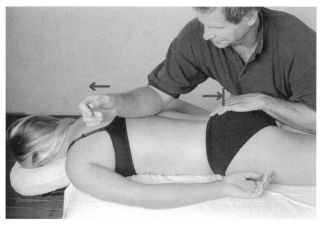

Figure 1-8

Cross-Fiber Strokes (DVD 2, 36:55)

Cross-fiber strokes are most commonly associated with a vigorous athletic massage, but are perfectly appropriate as an adjunct to deep tissue work if performed more slowly. Cross-fiber techniques are most often performed on the tendinous insertions of muscles, but are also useful in the muscle belly. The most common technique involves rolling the fingers over the tendon or muscle, back and forth, perpendicular to the fiber direction for two or three minutes. This should feel like rolling over a rope

Figure 1-9

that is resting on a hard surface. The purpose of cross-fiber work is to break up small adhesions or cross-fibers, but some research indicates that the primary benefit may be to stimulate collagen production. This is intense work that can be unpleasant for your client. Let your client know the difference between cross-fiber friction massage and the deep tissue work you have been performing. Explain that discomfort is normal and that some residual soreness may persist for a day. Applying ice afterwards is a good idea. Because of the intensity and vigorous nature of cross-fiber massage, I usually refer those clients who need extensive cross-fiber work to therapists who specialize in sports massage.

Separating Muscle Compartments

◎ This is extremely important and effective work. Perfecting muscle separation will drastically improve the effectiveness of your work and will result in a busier practice of return clients. Take the time to learn these skills.

Many muscles and tendons run parallel to each other and are designed to slide past each other during joint movement. For example, visualize the quadriceps muscles and the iliotibial band (IT band) above the knee. Beginning with the knee bent, as you straighten the knee, the hamstrings must lengthen while the quadriceps shorten. Between these two muscle groups, the IT band should be able to slide freely. If it adheres to either muscle group, it can be pulled anterior or posterior and create torsion at the knee.

Figure 1-10. Anatomy of the Quadriceps Muscles

The slightly different fiber directions of the vastus muscles in this drawing demonstrate the need for differentiation of muscle groups so that each muscle is able to properly exert its contractile force.

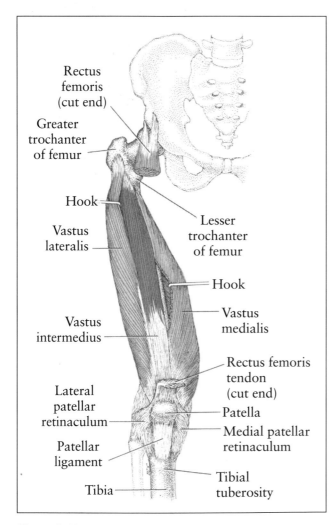

Rectus femoris (cut end)
Greater trochanter of femur
Hook
Vastus lateralis
Lesser trochanter of femur
Hook
Vastus intermedius
Vastus medialis
Rectus femoris tendon (cut end)
Patella
Medial patellar retinaculum
Lateral patellar retinaculum
Patellar ligament
Tibial tuberosity
Tibia

Figure 1-10

Many adjacent muscles exert slightly different angles of tension with movement throughout the entire body. Because of injury, holding patterns, inactivity, or immobility, these muscle compartments can become "glued" together and unable to slide. Precise and meticulous separation of these compartments is often the key to improving joint function and resolving nagging complaints that conventional treatment is unable to affect.

Figure 1-11. Separating Muscle Compartments (Deltoid or Pectoralis Major)

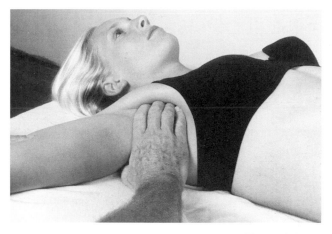

Sometimes, grabbing one muscle and rolling it away from its neighbor is a useful strategy. Moving the joint, either passively or asking the client to voluntarily move a joint greatly increases the effectiveness because one muscle will automatically begin to slide past its adjacent partner. Slowly let your fingers find an accessible entry between muscles and patiently follow the line separating the muscles.

Figure 1-11

Freeing Muscles from Entrapment (DVD 2, 41:38, 47:55 and 51:10)

Sometimes muscles are not "glued" to an adjacent muscle on the superficial surface of the body as described in the previous section but are adhered to deeper muscles, broad fascial sheets, or even to the bones. The following techniques are similar to those in the previous section, but are broader in scope and useful when you can not find a surface entry point to begin separating tissue. On yourself or your clients, palpate any long muscles such as the calf muscles, the quadriceps, hamstrings, or the biceps or triceps. Ideally, these muscles should only be attached to bones at their tendinous insertions. You should be able to *roll* muscles without feeling excessive binding to deeper layers. Pay attention to how free these areas feel in all your clients so that you have some standard to evaluate an area to determine if work is necessary. The techniques shown in Figures 1-12, 1-13, and 1-14 require patience; it may take several minutes to feel the entire muscle begin to roll away from a deeper layer.

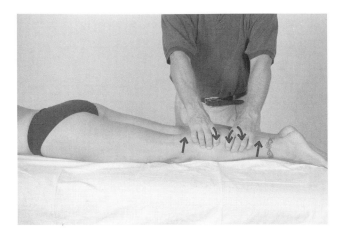

Figure 1-12

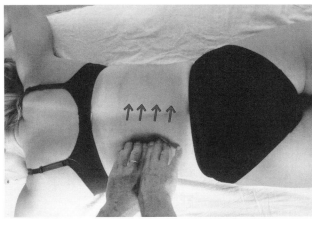

Figure 1-13

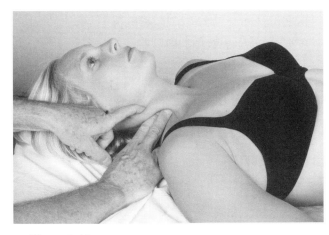

Figure 1-14

Figure 1-12. Lifting a Muscle from Deeper Restrictions (DVD 2, 34:31)

Grab the entire muscle with both hands. Slowly try to lift the belly of the muscle from the bone. Rotate the muscle both directions along its long axis like you would roll a pencil on a hard surface. Sometimes, it is effective to stretch the muscle in both directions also.

Figure 1-13. Mobilizing the Erector Spinae Muscles (DVD 2, 41:38)

Most techniques with the erectors emphasize either lengthening or softening this muscle group. However, some mobility in the lateral/medial direction is also important. Use the fingers of both hands to apply force along the border of the muscle and slowly push the muscle to the opposite side. Remember, you are not attempting to roll over the muscle as you would with cross-fiber techniques. You should visualize that you are snow-plowing the entire muscle to allow deviation from the sagittal plane.

Figure 1-14. Differentiating the Sternocleidomastoid Muscle (DVD 2, 45:30)

Notice on your clients how often the sternocleidomastoid muscle seems to be stuck to deeper layers of tissue. It may appear unusual to lift the muscle as the photo shows, but try it on yourself. It actually feels good.

Allowing a Muscle to Shorten

Many massage techniques focus on how to lengthen short muscles in order to facilitate greater range of motion for the joint. However, occasionally it seems that the muscle is unable to shorten effectively. For example, it is not uncommon for people to have difficulty dorsiflexing the ankle, even when the posterior compartment of the leg is not inhibiting motion by being too tight. The same phenomenon can occur at the wrist, the knee, or the hip. In the wrist or ankle, the motion can be impaired by the tendons adhering to the retinaculum. This could affect motion in either direction—if the tendons have adhered with the ankle in a flexed position, then it will be difficult to extend the ankle. If they are adhered in an extended joint position, then it will be difficult to flex the ankle.

Physiology texts explain how a muscle lengthens or shortens by the individual muscle cells or filaments sliding past each other in each direction. These fibers may adhere at a cellular level anywhere along a muscle, preventing either lengthening or shortening.

◎ When freeing a joint using the following techniques, it is much more effective to have the client actively contract the muscle while you anchor on the retinaculum in order to ascertain restrictions that prevent smooth movement.

Figure 1-15. How Fiber Restrictions Impede Proper Lengthening or Shortening of Tissue

When muscle cells can easily slide past each other, muscle movement is smooth and easy. If certain cells or muscle groups adhere to each other, a muscle may have difficulty shortening as well as lengthening. A buckling may occur on shortening, similar to a rug being wrinkled. If one section of a muscle behaves this way while other adjacent areas are able to either lengthen or shorten properly, it can cause torsion as the muscle contracts unevenly.

(See Figure 1-15 on page 36)

RESTRICTED TISSUE MOVEMENT

These figures represent the lengthening and contraction of different tissues. If areas of muscle or fascia are bound by adhesions or thickened tissue, they may be unable to smoothly contract or lengthen, causing impaired movement at joints.

RESTING LENGTH

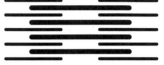

This figure represents muscle in a neutral position, ready to either be stretched or to contract.

LENGTHENING TISSUE

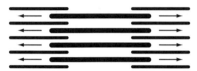

In this example, healthy tissue is being stretched. The different fibers are not impinged by adhesions and are able to easily slide past each other without any torsion.

SHORTENING TISSUE

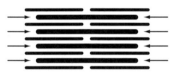

The absence of adhesions allows the fibers to smoothly and evenly contract without any interference.

RESTRICTED LENGTHENING

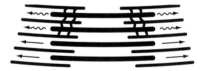

The fibers at the top of this representation are unable to slide past each other because of adhesions or other restrictions, while the fibers at the bottom are free to slide properly. This disparity causes the tissue to lengthen in an uneven manner which can cause strain on joints.

RESTRICTED SHORTENING

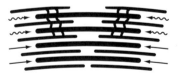

In this example, the upper fibers are adhered to each other and unable to properly shorten or contract while the lower fibers are able to slide past each other easily. As in the Restricted Lengthening example, this tissue will contract in an uneven manner and cause torsion and strain on joints.

Figure 1-15

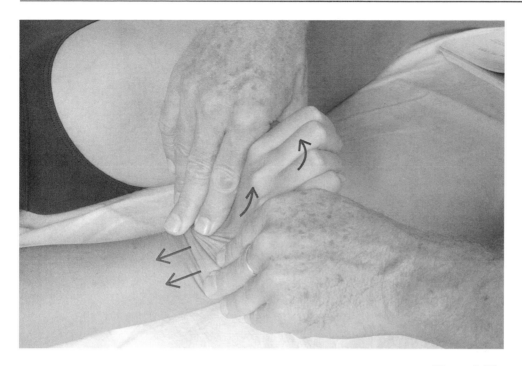

Figure 1-16a

Figures 1-16 a and b. Facilitating Shortening of Muscles (DVD 2, 20:51 and 23:29)

While having client flex the wrist or ankle, facilitate shortening of the muscle or free restrictions in the retinaculum by applying force in the direction of shortening wherever you feel tissue bunching. This technique will be even more effective if you have the client actively contract the muscle rather than remaining passive while you move the joint.

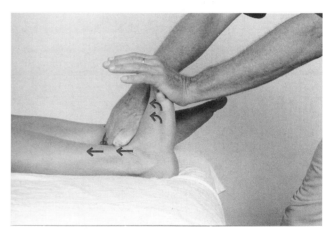

Figure 1-16b

Note: Notice the difference between these techniques and facilitating lengthening movement by working in the direction of muscle lengthening (as shown previously in Figure 1-9).

One of the most common questions I receive concerns when to use "facilitated lengthening" strokes that apply force in the direction of muscle lengthening, and when to use anchor and stretch strokes. There are no hard-and-fast rules, but the majority of your strokes will be lengthening and are most useful when an entire muscle is tight and short. Anchor and stretch strokes are most useful when you find isolated adhesions that need to be released, and are usually performed more slowly as you wait for the muscle to "melt." Anchoring on the localized spasm or adhesion and very slowly stretching the muscle by moving the joint through its range of motion will allow you to pinpoint your energy at a specific point as you wait for release. Remember that you will not be moving your anchor by sliding over the tissue. Imagine that you are grabbing a knot in a rubber band as you stretch the muscle away from that area.

Chapter Two

General Techniques

◎ The focus of this chapter will be proper use of the tools at your disposal—the fingers, knuckles, fist, forearm, and elbow. Once you become comfortable using these techniques, later chapters will provide specific treatment strategies for different parts of the body and will explain in more detail how to perform the movements here shown as examples.

The Hierarchy of Power

It is ironic that the more tightness in a client's body, the greater the natural tendency for the therapist to strain to remove that tightness. It is difficult to remove tension by imposing tension and yet strain is inevitable when attempting to use thumbs and fingers for deep work. Most massage therapists have had more practice, and therefore, have more confidence working with their fingers and thumbs. Because they are so comfortable and confident in using their hands for all work, many are reluctant to use other more powerful tools that would enable them to work with greater ease and effectiveness and with less strain. The reality is that for deep work, few people have the strength to do all the work with their fingers. Learning to use the knuckles, fist, forearm, and elbow will allow you to do work with less effort, thus protecting your own body and enabling you to release more tension in the client's body.

As a general rule, there is a hierarchy of power and effectiveness as one progresses up the chain from using the fingers up to the elbow. If you find yourself straining using your fingers, try using your knuckles. If the knuckles are not providing enough power or are concentrating force in too narrow an area, the fist is often effective. Use of the forearm allows you even more power and has the flexibility of allowing use of the relatively hard bony surface of the ulna or the fleshier undersurface of the forearm. If you wish to concentrate your energy into a smaller area, the elbow then becomes your most effective tool.

These alternatives are not limited to Deep Tissue Massage. They offer a wide range of tactile sensations for the client and enable the therapist to utilize energy efficiently for shallow or subtle work. With practice, you will feel as confident in your touch working with your elbows as with your hands.

Just Say "No" to Thumbs (DVD 1, 1:05:03)

T HE THUMBS ARE A WONDERFUL TOOL FOR MASSAGE, but they are not intended for extended periods of use performing deep work. Tendonitis or, even worse, arthritis of the thumb is one of the most common and debilitating injuries to massage therapists. Sometimes experienced therapists are laying the groundwork for serious injury for years before symptoms surface. Once symptoms arise, it may be too late to reverse the damage. I have known several excellent massage therapists who had to change careers because of thumb pain.

Examine an anatomy text to see how the thumb articulates with the metacarpals and you will see how precarious the joint is. The following photographs demonstrate the hazards of using the thumbs for hard work. Break your habits of using the thumbs for deep work and you will have the benefit of their pain-free use for effleurage for the rest of your career.

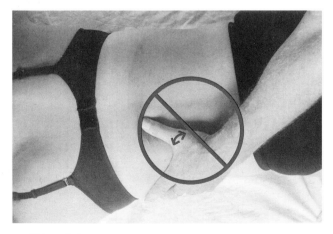

Figure 2-1. Improper Use of the Thumbs

If you keep your wrist in a neutral position, notice the shearing force on the thumb joint, which can cause arthritis by wearing away the articular cartilage. Tendonitis of the muscles that flex the thumb may also result.

Figure 2-1

Figure 2-2. Compromised Wrist Mechanics When Using Thumbs

In this photograph, force is applied with the thumb in a straight line with the forearm in an attempt to alleviate the shearing stress shown in the previous example. However, it is clear that the wrist is compromised and will be vulnerable to strain and injury.

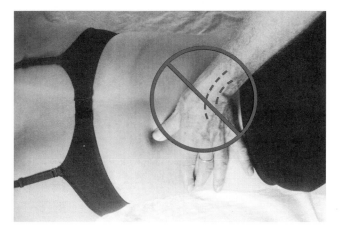

Proper Use of the Fingers (DVD 1, 52:20)

Figure 2-2

THE FINGERS WILL TAKE CONSIDERABLE TIME AND PRACTICE to be strong enough for very deep work, but unless you are double-jointed, after while they will gain strength and can be the most sensitive tool you have for deep work. Always keep the fingers slightly bent and work primarily with the soft pads. Keep the wrists in a neutral position so that they are not bent into flexion/extension or inversion/eversion. Any time the fingers begin to hyperextend, shake, or show other signs of fatigue, utilize another tool such as knuckles or the elbow. If your hands are not strong enough, work with one hand over the other to add support.

Figure 2-3. Proper Use of the Fingers

Notice that wrists are in a neutral position in relation to flexion/extension and inversion/eversion. Fingers are relaxed and slightly flexed. Apply force at an oblique angle and visualize stretching tissue rather than just squeezing or sliding over the skin because too much lubricant is used.

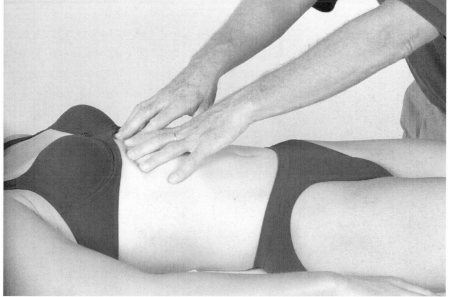

Figure 2-3

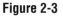

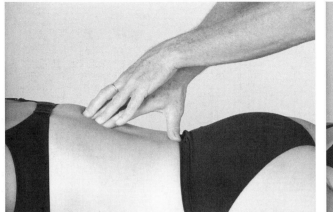

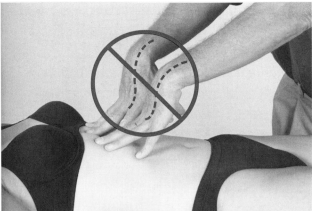

Figure 2-4   **Figure 2-5**

Figure 2-4. Reinforcing Fingers by Using Both Hands
Working with one hand over the other will provide more depth with less effort.

Figure 2-5. Improper Use of the Fingers
Notice that the wrist is flexed and fingers are hyper-extended and tense.

Use of Knuckles Instead of Thumbs (DVD 1, 1:08:04)

THE THUMBS ARE A VERSATILE AND IMPORTANT OPTION for massage strokes such as effleurage. However, overuse injuries to thumbs can end your career as a massage therapist. In order to save your thumbs from injury when working deeply, the knuckles offer the most effective substitute. Often, they will actually feel better to the client and will save your energy, enabling you to give more massages. In the following figures notice that the nondominant hand is always involved in helping to accomplish the goals. In the first case, the left hand is opening the client's hand, in the second it is stretching the foot into plantar flexion, and in the third, it is stabilizing the foot.

When using the knuckles it is very important that the wrist and the joint between the metacarpals and phalanges be straight. If either of these joints collapses, most of your power is lost and the hand becomes vulnerable to injury. The different lengths of the fingers necessitate using only one or two knuckles rather than all four. Rotation of the shoulder joint rather than the wrist is the primary method of changing the angle of use.

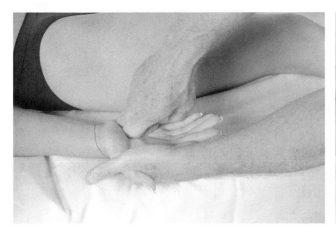

Figure 2-6

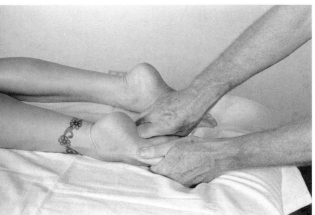

Figure 2-7

Figure 2-6. Use of Knuckles Instead of Thumbs

If the therapist were to use knuckles instead of thumbs on just the hands and feet, the use of thumbs could be cut by one-third to one-half.

Figure 2-7. Use of Knuckles on the Plantar Surface of the Foot

The therapist can plantarflex the ankle with his left hand to provide stretch to tight tissue while working towards the calcaneous with the right knuckles.

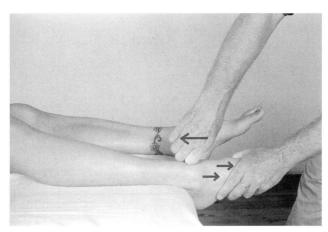

Figure 2-8

Figure 2-8. Knuckles—Ankle Retinaculum

Notice the stability in the wrist and knuckles while the left hand manipulates the foot.

Figure 2-9. Knuckles— Proper Rotation of the Arm

When using long strokes such as working in the spinal groove, many students find that the knuckles are most easily used by internally rotating the entire arm so the thumb is down and the palm is facing away.

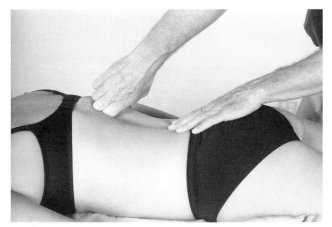

Figure 2-9

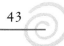

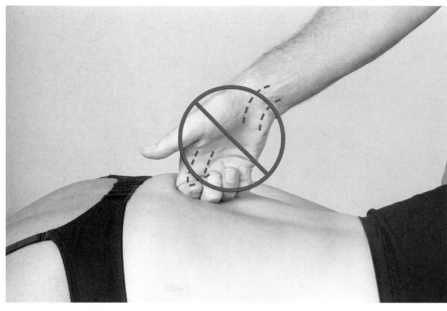

Figure 2-10. Knuckles—Improper Arm Rotation

Notice that with the thumb up and the arm rotated externally, there is a tendency for the fingers and wrist to collapse.

Figure 2-10

An Example: Knuckles and Fingers— Occiput, Forehead, Temple

Many people are surprised how much tension lies in the muscles and fascia of the skull. Very slow work on sensitive or tight areas can help alleviate headache symptoms and release the strain from the muscles of facial expression. Specific techniques will be demonstrated in later sections, but beginning to practice now will make that approach easier to assimilate.

Figure 2-11. Working with the Cranium

Precaution: Never work in the sphenoid area of the temple.

Figure 2-12. Knuckles for Forehead Work

Using the soft aspect of your knuckles can feel very good to your client to release tension in the frontalis and other muscles of facial expression.

Figure 2-13. Knuckles for the Mastoid Process

Rotate the head for easy access to the mastoid process and occipital ridge.

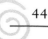

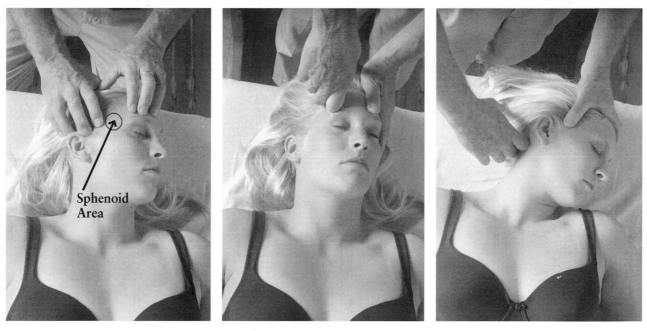

Figure 2-11   **Figure 2-12**   **Figure 2-13**

Use of the Fist (DVD 1, 1:19:31)

THE *fist* IS ACTUALLY THE USE OF THE FOUR KNUCKLES between the metacarpals and phalanges. The fingers are not contracted into a tight fist, but should be loosely extended, and the thumb should be relaxed and not gripped by the fingers. The fist is very useful as a relatively broad working surface for work on most fleshy areas of the body. In most cases, the elbow should be extended when using the fist, or it should be bent and braced against your pelvis. It is also useful for working in a client's pelvic area when working on the gluteals from above. Having the table low or climbing onto the table enables you to use gravity and your own weight to apply pressure downward. It is also very useful to use the fist in an oblique direction on the arms, legs, back, and on the hands and feet in place of using your thumbs.

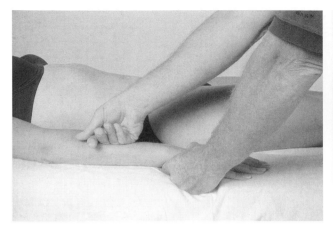

Figure 2-14a

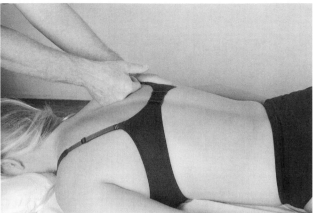

Figure 2-14b

Figures 2-14 a and b. Proper Use of the Fist

The most important consideration is to be sure that the wrist is in a neutral position. It should not be in a position of flexion or extension, or of inversion or eversion. Many students initially feel awkward in learning to use the fist. Most often you will feel most comfortable if you turn your palm up into a position similar to shaking hands.

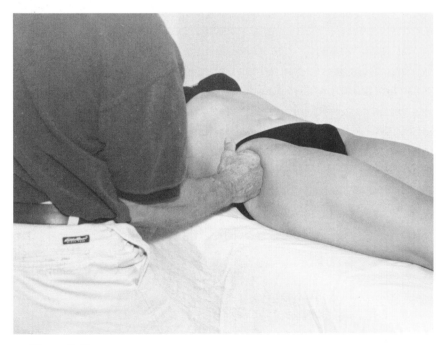

Figure 2-15. Bracing the Elbow Against Your Hip

In this case, the elbow is braced against the hip so that the energy is provided by the therapist's body weight transmitted through the pelvis rather than by muscular effort.

Figure 2-15

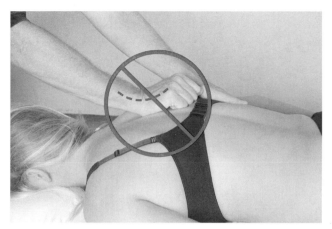

Figure 2-16a

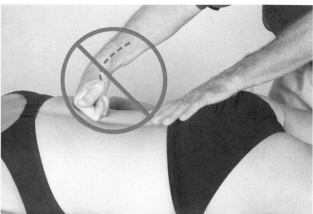

Figure 2-16b

Figures 2-16 a and b. Improper Use of the Fist

The most common error in using the fist is to apply oblique pressure with the palm down, which puts strain on the wrist joint as it moves into extension. However, with the wrist in a flexed position, if the fingers are clenched too tightly, the thumb is tense, and the wrist is compromised, then strain is spreads up the entire arm.

Figure 2-17. The Fist and Body Mechanics

When using the fist in long body strokes, it is important to be far enough away from the subject that your arm is relatively straight. The energy should either be oblique and directed from your feet, or your body should be directly above where you are working so that gravity provides the force. Be careful to not overuse the muscles of the shoulder girdle.

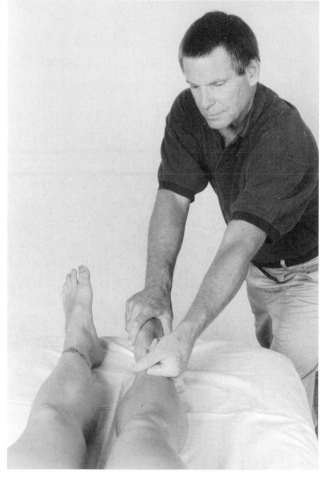

Figure 2-17

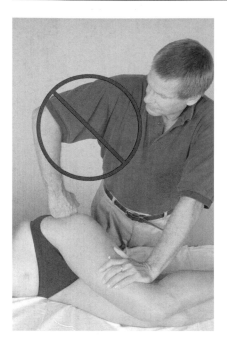

Figure 2-18

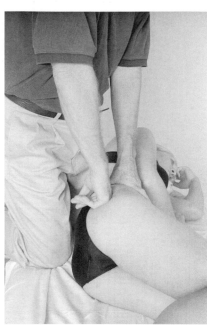

Figure 2-19

Figure 2-18. Improper Body Mechanics and the Fist

Notice the strain in the therapist's right shoulder and upper arm because the table is too high.

Figure 2-19. Adapting Body Mechanics for Proper Use of the Fist

To properly use gravity, climbing on the table will remove the strain to the therapist's shoulder and arms. Notice that the palm of the hand is facing the therapist's body.

Use of the Forearm (DVD 2, 0:22)

T HE FOREARM IS A USEFUL TOOL when you need a broader surface than the elbow or when the wrist is showing strain. It is also a good way to exert force vertically downward when the table is too high to properly use gravity by using the hands with the elbow extended. Depending on the type of tissue you are working on, you may use the soft, fleshy aspect of the forearm, or you may rotate your forearm externally to utilize the ulnar surface. Remember to exert force close to the elbow for efficient transmission of energy and to keep your wrist and hand relaxed. When applying force obliquely, remember to use your legs as the primary source of energy rather than your shoulder. The forearm is extremely helpful virtually anywhere on the client's body below the cervicals.

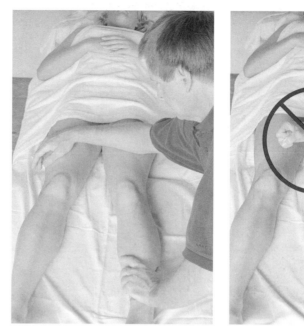

Figure 2-20. Proper Use of the Forearm

Figure 2-20

Figure 2-21

Force is applied close to the elbow rather than near the wrist. The elbow is at approximately a ninety-degree angle so that the biceps and triceps can relax and no energy is lost in the transmission of force. The wrist and hand are relaxed.

Figure 2-21. Improper Use of the Forearm

Notice that the contact point is too near the wrist, requiring upper arm tension to hold the elbow stable. This tension is apparent in the tight fist; it is difficult to remove tension from a client's body if your own body is tense.

Figure 2-22. Forearm Use on the Quadriceps

The forearm can be used moving in a proximal or distal direction. Be sure to exert pressure obliquely and not to press directly into the bone. The forearm is useful for broad work to dissipate deep muscle tension, but is not precise enough to separate quadriceps compartments. Be sure to work slowly and not to compress the patella. Most work will be in the direction of the muscle because there is not enough control for cross-fiber work.

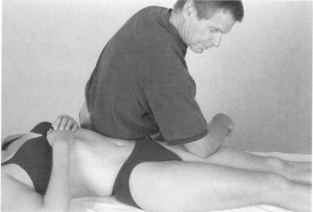

Figure 2-22

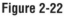

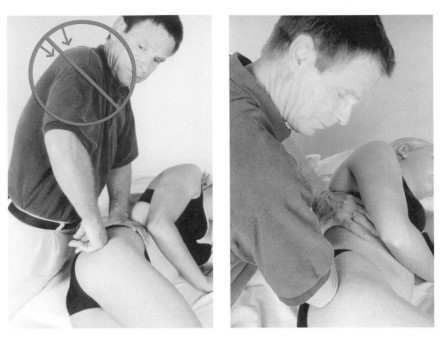

Figure 2-23   Figure 2-24

Figure 2-23. Improper Body Mechanics and the Fist

Note the strain to the therapist's upper body when using the fist. Climbing on the table would provide better leverage, and Figure 2-24 offers yet another alternative.

Figure 2-24. Changing Tools Instead of Changing Your Position

If you find a particular stroke is not working well for you, it may be easier to change to a different technique instead of drastically altering your position. If climbing on the table is inconvenient, switching to the elbow or forearm allows the therapist to use his own weight rather than using excess muscular effort.

Use of the Elbow (DVD 2, 9:32)

BECAUSE OF THE BROAD SURFACE through which force is distributed, the forearm is sometimes inappropriate to focus energy at a deep level without strain to your own body. When this is the case, the elbow is needed to focus force in a smaller area. Although many massage therapists are tentative about utilizing this tool, use of the elbow is actually one of the easiest techniques to learn. There are none of the problems of instability encountered with fingers, knuckles, or fists. Anywhere below the client's cervicals, the elbow can be substituted in almost any situation where the thumbs are used. The elbow should be bent at approximately ninety degrees with the forearm and hand relaxed. Although it is much easier to push away from your body with both the forearm and elbow, they may also be pulled towards your own body in a raking movement.

Experiment to find which arm position works best for you; some therapists find that having the humerus internally rotated works more efficiently while others prefer to externally rotate the humerus. Placing the elbow between the thumb and forefinger of the opposite hand will add stability and prevent it from slipping in areas where very specific force is needed.

◎ Caution: Apply force distal to the olecranon process of your elbow. The ulnar nerve is vulnerable directly above the elbow and may become inflamed if it is stimulated.

Figure 2-25. The Elbow for Detailed Work (Spine)

The elbow is a fine tool for working virtually any place on the back. It can be used instead of using the thumbs for very precise work next to the spine with the erector spinae muscles. Elbows can also be utilized from a slightly different angle for broader strokes with the larger back muscles such as the latissimus dorsi and trapezius muscles. Notice how the therapist's body weight is used to supply the force for the stroke. The elbow can almost always accomplish the most work with the least effort, but because it is such a powerful tool, take particular care near the floating ribs, which are more vulnerable to deep pressure.

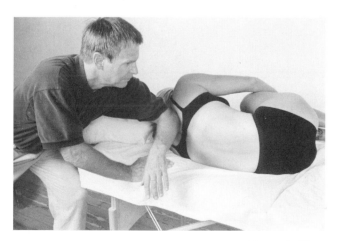

Figure 2-25

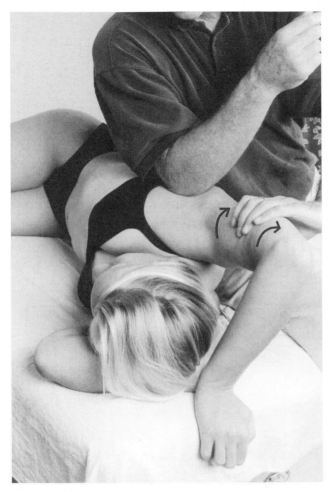

Figure 2-26

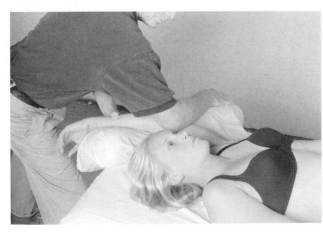

Figure 2-27

Figure 2-26. Freeing the Scapula with the Elbow

Externally rotating the humerus and abducting the arm will open the area around your client's lateral scapula.

General Strategies

Placing Muscles in a Stretched Position (DVD 2, 53:29)

Many of the following strategies will be explained in more detail in later sections. These are a few examples to demonstrate methods of working on muscles that are in a stretched position. Have fun inventing stretches of your own.

Figure 2-27. Stretching the Triceps (DVD 2, 1:06:54)

By placing the client's arm above the head, the triceps group is lengthened, enabling a neurological release so that the muscles will actually rest at a longer length after the massage. Your forearm, fist, etc. can then be used to work the arm. Flexing the client's elbow will increase the stretch to the triceps.

Precautions: If the client has had a shoulder separation or if mobility is limited, do not use this positioning. If mobility is slightly impaired, the arm can be supported by a pillow.

Figure 2-28. Stretching the Teres Muscles—Supine

While the client is supine, stretching the arm above the head will open the lateral scapula to enable work on the subscapularis and the teres group.

Figure 2-29. Internal Arm Rotation—Prone

Placing the arm in different positions will stretch different muscles. By abducting the humerus with the palm up, the arm is placed into internal rotation. The internal rotation will stretch the teres minor (an external rotator of the humerus) while the abduction of the arm will stretch both the teres major and minor.

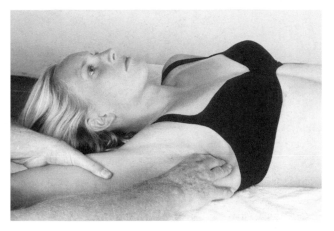

Figure 2-28

Figure 2-30. Lumber Rotation Stretch—Prone

Use one hand to rotate the pelvis in one direction while working in the other direction with the other hand or forearm. Specific stretches will be covered in later sections; the main point is to feel free to place the body in rotational stretches to free vertebral articulations and stretch muscles.

Contraindications: Avoid rotational stretches if the client is experiencing back pain.

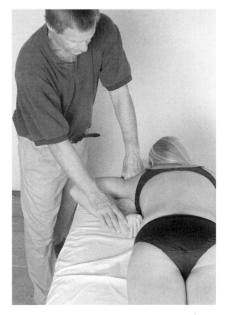

Figure 2-29

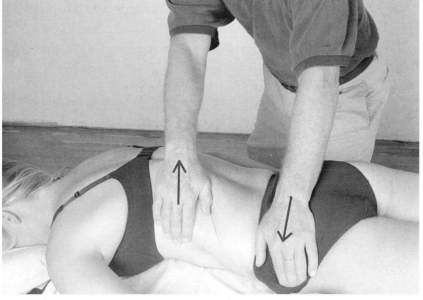

Figure 2-30

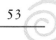

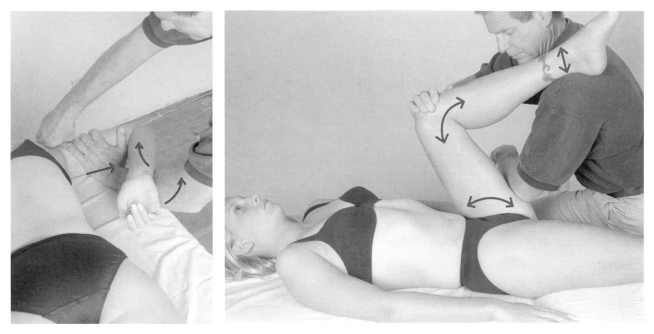

Figure 2-31   **Figure 2-32**

Figure 2-31. Internal Arm Rotation—Prone

This position is similar to that used in Figure 2-29 to work on the teres major, teres minor, and other rotator cuff muscles, except that by placing your arm under the forearm and grasping over the humerus, many movement variations are possible. You may distract the shoulder joint, abduct or adduct the arm, and can move the humerus from internal to external rotation to work different muscles in various lengths of stretch.

Figure 2-32. Supine Hamstring Work (DVD 2, 1:01:55)

The entire length of the hamstrings can be worked in this position. The amount of knee and hip flexion will determine the degree of stretch to the hamstrings and is determined by the left hand. Pushing the knee to increase hip flexion will stretch the hamstrings near their origin at the pelvis, while elevating your shoulder will straighten the knee to stretch the distal aspects of the muscle.

Making Use of the Side-Lying Position (DVD 2, 1:09:11)

Therapists are often hesitant to take the short time necessary to place clients on their sides for work. However, it is an excellent strategy to approach some areas that are difficult to access in the prone or supine positions. Clients almost always enjoy this alternative. It is extremely useful if your client is experiencing acute low back distress because while you are working you can find the neutral pelvic position that is pain-free. These techniques will be covered in more detail in later sections of this manual. For now, some basic techniques will be shown to enable you to begin practicing.

◎ Side-lying work is such an important adjunct to your work, that a few more words are necessary to attempt to insure that you take the time to develop skills working in this position. I've had countless students say that learning to work in this manner has totally altered and increased the success of their practice. One student reported that a client had been sampling work from many therapists while searching for someone to see on a regular basis. When this student worked on the man in the side-lying position, he immediately said that he had never experienced work in this manner, and that he didn't need to look any further for a regular therapist. He began receiving two ninety-minute sessions a week. This student attributes an increase of over seven thousand dollars a year from this client alone to his strategy of placing his client in the side-lying position.

Throughout my years of teaching Deep Tissue Massage to therapists, I've found that students are invariably excited by how effective and fun side-lying work is. They leave class with enthusiastic plans to use their new skills. However, when class resumes the next week, only a few students indicate that they actually used the techniques. It didn't take long to determine that their hesitancy could be traced to their original training. Most beginning massage classes pay lip service to side-lying work, and then only as a technique to be used with pregnant women. We learn massage like it is a chess game with only one move: begin with the clients in prone position and approximately half way through, have them turn over; or begin in supine position and turn to prone. Many classes overemphasize the "blissed-out" disassociative aspects of massage to the exclusion of other therapeutic goals. Some therapists have the misconception that it would be disruptive or even irritating to disturb a relaxed client by asking her to turn on her side. However, you will be surprised how willing your clients are to try new positions and how quickly they will return to a relaxed state.

We often limit ourselves in many aspects of our lives by unexamined mindsets or habits. If you find that you are hesitant to try side-lying or any other techniques you learn in this book or other classes, take some time to examine your resistance. Are you uncomfortable during the learning period that is a necessary stage of mastering new skills? Are you performing massage in a rote, repetitious manner? Are you hesitant to assert yourself by instructing clients to move to a different position? Are you wasting time by working too long in areas that only need brief attention so that you don't have the time to give proper attention to areas of deep tension, or to move a client into a different position? Do you feel free to inform your clients that a longer massage would offer them much greater benefit (as well as more income for yourself)? Using the side-lying position will change the way you look at massage. Try it!

Working the Adductors in the Side-Lying Position

The adductors are one of the most underworked parts of the body in massage. Part of the reason for this is the difficulty in finding a comfortable and secure position in the supine position. Having the client in side-lying position enables the client to feel less vulnerable in the groin area and offers a multitude of options concerning hip flexion/extension and knee flexion/extension. Work with fingers, knuckles, fist, and forearm are all appropriate.

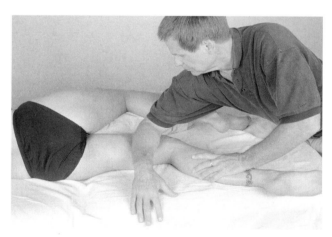

Figure 2-33. Side-Lying Adductor Work
(DVD 2, 1:10:48)

Note that the opposite leg is flexed forward and supported by a bolster in order to minimize rotational stress to the lumbar region. Goals can be to lengthen the adductors or to separate and better define the various components of the medial leg.

Figure 2-33

Other Uses of Side-Lying

Figure 2-34. Side-Lying "Window Wiper"

To add stability for broad strokes on the back, you can anchor your hand on the table and rotate your forearm back and forth similar to the movement of wiper blades on an automobile. The distance at which you place your hand from your client's back will determine how sharp or broad the stroke will be. Keep wrist flexion to a minimum in order to not strain your wrist.

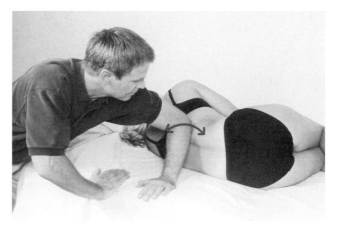

Figure 2-34

Figure 2-35. Side-Lying Hip Work

This is one of the most effective ways to free the entire lateral pelvis, rotators, and quadratus lumborum. The upper leg can be in many positions. With the knee forward, muscles of the posterior compartment are put on a stretch. The anterior muscles such as tensor fascia latae may be extended with the leg pulled down and back. Support the upper leg with bolsters as needed. Extending the leg downward as far as possible will open the quadratus area. Specific techniques will be explained in later sections.

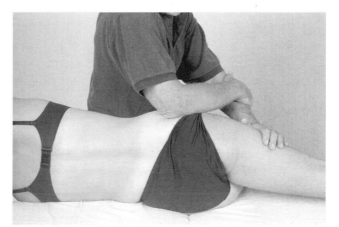

Figure 2-35

Precautions: Work gently around the floating ribs and kidneys and be cautious to not apply direct pressure on the sciatic nerve where it descends down the leg beneath the external leg rotators.

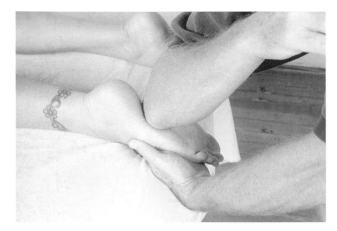

Figure 2-36

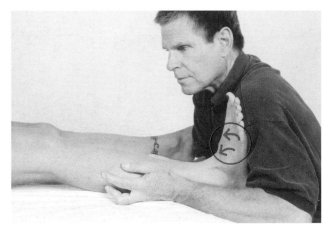

Figure 2-37

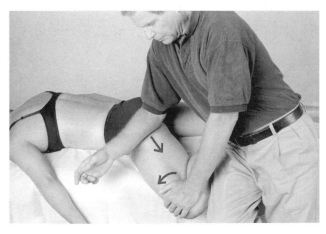

Figure 2-38

Using a Full Range of Alternatives in Position

Figure 2-36. Elbow for the Plantar Surface of the Foot

This is another substitute for using the thumbs. Notice that the left hand supports the foot.

Figure 2-37. Supine Calf Work

Note that the therapist can dorsiflex the ankle by pushing his shoulder against the instep of the foot. This enables the calf to be stretched while it is being massaged.

The lateral compartment of the upper leg is often ignored in a general massage but work in this area can offer great relief for a variety of complaints, including low back pain and knee pain. The primary interest now is in positioning your client in order to address this area. Be sure that any force is applied in an oblique direction rather than directly against the femur. Generally, work in a direction away from the acetabulum to decompress the hip joint. Detailed directions for working on this area will be covered later in the manual.

Figure 2-38. Prone Abductor Work

This method is most easily incorporated into a short massage when there is not enough time to do side-lying work.

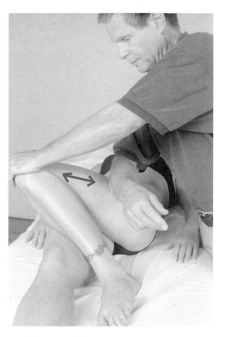

Figure 2-39. Supine Abductor Work

This is another nonspecific way of loosening the iliotibial band that is easily incorporated into a massage when you are not doing side-lying work. However, working away from the hip joint can place rotational strain on the back. For this reason, it is advisable to work in a downward direction towards the hip joint, even though this does not offer the benefit of decompressing the joint.

Figure 2-40. Side-Lying Abductor Work (DVD 3, 1:02:25)

Of the three positions, this is the most versatile; the ability to flex or extend the hip and to flex or extend the knee allows for many variations in stretching individual muscles and increasing joint mobility.

Figure 2-39

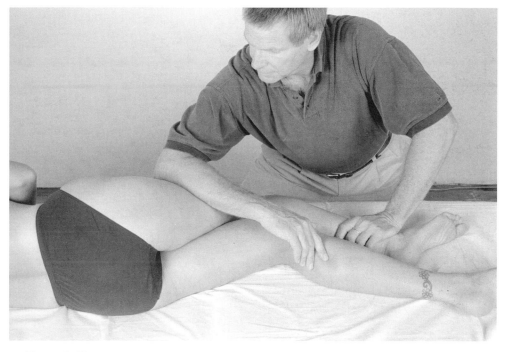

Figure 2-40

Chapter Three

Specific Strategies

Now that you are familiar with the major tools you will use in Deep Tissue Massage, we will combine the broad theories of deep work from Chapter One and the general techniques for use of knuckles, fist, forearm, and the elbow offered in Chapter Two into specific strategies for use on different areas of the body. Please feel free to experiment to adapt these suggestions to your own personal style. You may feel more comfortable using your elbow where a photograph demonstrates use of the knuckles. You may not feel comfortable or confident using your elbow as shown in an example and will want to use your fist. Be creative and have fun experimenting!

Working with the Foot and Lower Leg (DVD 3, 1:22)

STRUCTURAL WORK ON THE FOOT will have a dramatic effect upon the success of your practice by differentiating your work from the usual strokes designed to give temporary relief to tired or painful feet. With practice, you can learn to give freedom to immobile joints and dramatically improve the transmission of stress through the body by providing better balance in the feet.

High and Low Arches

Figure 3-1. The Arches of the Foot

Would you work the same way on the feet shown in Figures 3-2 and 3-3? Notice how the structure of feet can have very different effects upon how the

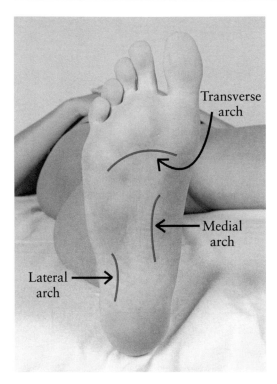

Figure 3-1

shock of impact when walking is transmitted through the legs and the pelvis.

Figure 3-2. Feet with High Arches

The high medial arch that shifts weight to the outside of the foot will transmit stress up the outside of the legs to the hips. Working to create flexibility in the medial arch will enable the foot to land more evenly on the ground and transmit weight more uniformly up the legs.

Figure 3-3. Feet with Low Arches

It is more difficult to alter structure in the low arched foot because this condition is primarily a result of too much mobility in the medial arch due to bone structure or loose ligaments. Stretching tissue in the medial arch could exacerbate this hypermobility, but working to mobilize the lateral arch can mitigate some of the stress that is being shifted to the medial arch. As the lateral arch becomes more flexible, it will absorb shock instead of shifting weight to the inside of the foot. Notice how the stress of standing or the

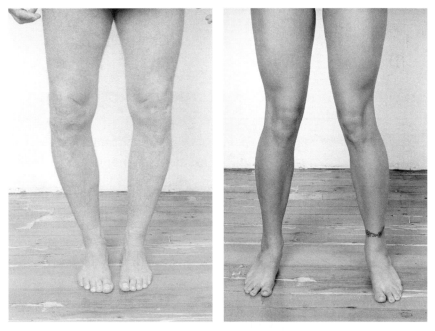

Figure 3-2   **Figure 3-3**

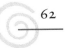

shock of walking will be transmitted to the medial legs, through the medial knee and up to the pubic symphysis.

In both these cases, an understanding of the feet can give important clues about where your client will be experiencing tension or pain. For example, you would not have to palpate tissue in the legs to know that someone with high arches and bow legs would probably be tight in the peroneals, the IT band and the lateral hips. Conversely, someone with flat feet and knock-knees will appreciate work on the adductors.

Figure 3-4. Anatomy of the Foot Flexors and Extensors (DVD 3, 5:55)

Note the muscles of foot movement and the importance of specific focused work on individual muscles rather than broad general strokes.

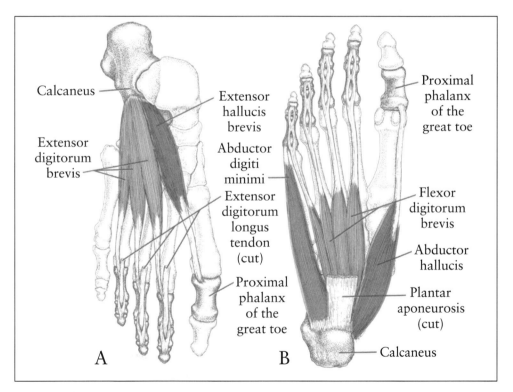

Figure 3-4

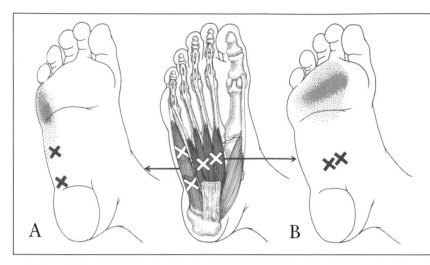

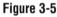

Figure 3-5. Anatomy of Foot Flexors with Trigger Points

This drawing clarifies the relationship between the muscles and the fleshy covering of the foot. Notice the trigger point referral points to painful areas of the foot.

Figure 3-6. Anatomy of the Layers of Lower Leg Muscles

Notice the different layers of the muscles of the lower leg and the separation between the flexors and extensors of the foot. Also note the location of the major nerves and blood vessels. The depth of these structures protects them from injury and allows Deep Tissue Massage to be performed in relative safety.

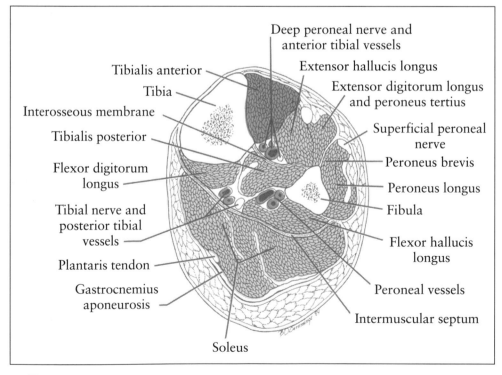

The Plantar Surface of the Foot (3, 11:11)

When working with the plantar surface of the foot, have a clear intention of what you want to accomplish. Do you want to lengthen the medial arch, to widen or improve flexion in the transverse arch, to create better movement between the metatarsals, to mobilize the calcaneus? As good as kneading the feet with Swedish techniques feels, working structurally to improve function and mobility of the foot can have lasting results and will be appreciated by your clients.

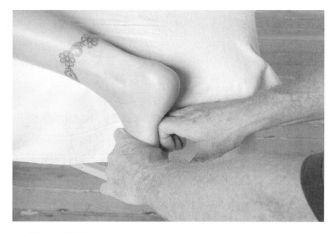

Figure 3-7

Figure 3-7. Moving the Leg to Allow Flexion of the Ankle

While working, use your other hand to invert, evert, plantarflex, dorsiflex, or in other ways increase mobility in the foot. Supporting the foot with a bolster, moving the leg to have the foot hanging over the side of the table, or having the client slide down so that the feet hang over the edge of the table all allow manipulation of the foot and ankle to stretch tissue and mobilize joints.

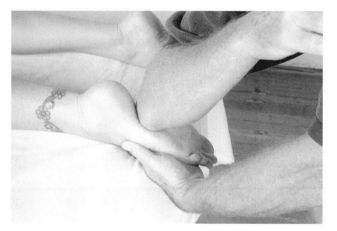

Figure 3-8

Figure 3-8. Elbow for Specific Work on the Lateral Arch

The elbow is an excellent tool to save your thumbs.

Figure 3-9. Mobilizing the Calcaneous with the Fingers

While client is supine, flex the knee so the foot lies flat on the table. In this example, the calcaneus is being mobilized in a posterior direction with the bottom hand. This technique could be called "snowplowing." Rather than sliding over tissue, visualize grabbing tissue and pushing it posterior, along with the calcaneous. You may

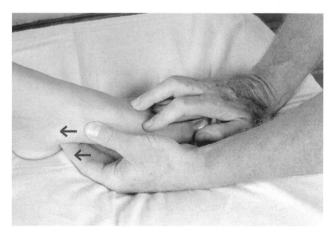

Figure 3-9

also use your fingers to widen the foot above or below, or pull tissue towards yourself to create length in the foot. Be aware of the mobility of the individual metatarsal bones, generally working to accomplish shearing mobility between each bone.

Figure 3-10. Anatomy of the Tibialis Anterior Muscle

In addition to dorsiflexing the foot, the tibialis anterior also supports the medial arch. For clients with high arches, stretching and relaxing this muscle can be important to allow the medial arch to relax. Notice the ankle retinaculum: if it is fibrosed, it can impede smooth flexion of the ankle and disrupt the efficient action of muscle contraction.

Origin: *Lateral condyle of tibia*

Insertion: *Media and plantar surface of medial cuneiform bone and base of first metatarsal*

Action: *To maintain standing balance, foot dorsiflexion and supination*

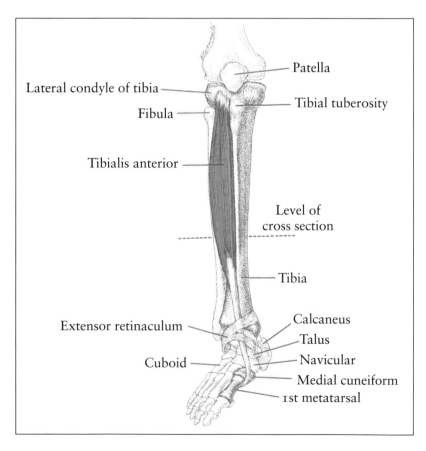

Figure 3-10

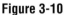

Figure 3-11. Anatomy of the Peroneals

An everted foot may be a result of short or fibrosed peroneals.
Origin: Fibula and adjacent intermuscular septa
Insertion: First metatarsal and medial cuneiform bones
Action: To evert foot and assist in plantar flexion of foot

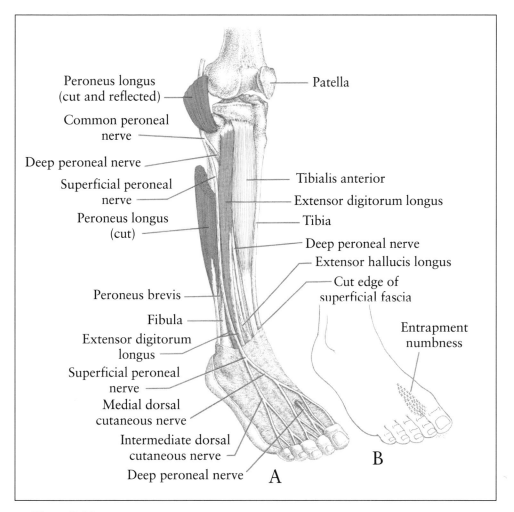

Figure 3-11

Ankle Retinaculum

The ankle retinaculum (see Figure 3-10, page 66) is an important structure that is often neglected in massage. Freeing this area enables increased dorsiflexion and plantarflexion and proper tracking of the ankle.

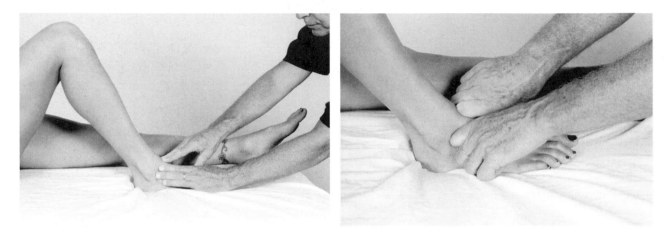

Figure 3-12a

Figure 3-12b

Figures 3-12 a and b. Working with the Ankle Retinaculum

Use of fingers, knuckles, forearm, and even the elbows is effective. Soften fibrous areas around both malleoli and at the junction between the tibia and talus bones. Use your other hand to move the ankle through its complete range of motion while you are working.

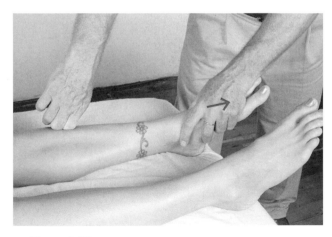

Figure 3-13

Anterior Leg (DVD 3, 14:52)

Figure 3-13. Knuckle Work on the Anterior Tibia

Work on the lateral side of the tibia in either direction. Passively extend the foot and look for areas where the tissue does not move freely. Work these areas with the fist, forearm, knuckles or even the elbow while moving the ankle to stretch the tissue.

Figure 3-14. Fist Work on the Anterior Tibia in the Prone Position

Notice the proper use of gravity with the therapist kneeling on the table. This position is par-

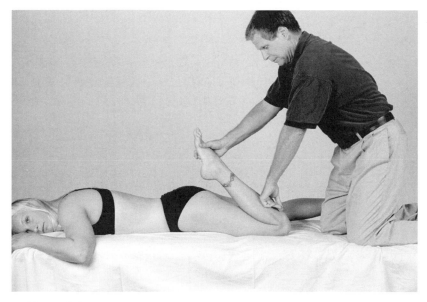

Figure 3-14

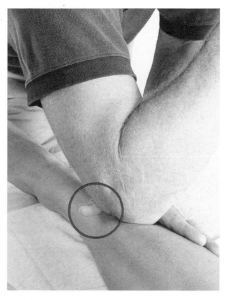

Figure 3-15

ticularly effective to localize stretch just below the knee.

Figure 3-15. Elbow Work on the Anterior Tibia

The elbow can be an effective tool for softening or freeing the tibialis anterior from the tibia. Note the use of the left hand to stabilize the elbow between the thumb and index finger.

Figure 3-16. Anatomy of the Gastrocnemius Muscle

Notice the two heads of the gastrocnemius. Depending upon the support of the foot, the different heads may have very different degrees of tightness.

Origin: *Posterior femur*
Insertion: *Calcaneus*
Action: *Plantar flexion of foot*

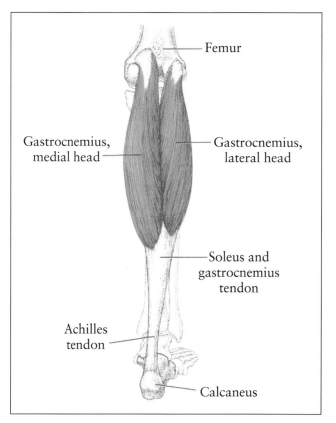

Figure 3-16

Figure 3-17. Anatomy of the Soleus Muscle

Because the soleus lies deep to the gastrocnemius, it is sometimes necessary to soften the gastrocnemius by flexing the knee or plantarflexing the ankle to enable the therapist to penetrate to the deeper soleus. The plantaris muscle may be a factor in posterior knee pain.

> Origin: Posterior tibia and fibula
>
> Insertion: Calcaneus
>
> Action: Plantar flexion of foot—particularly when knee is flexed

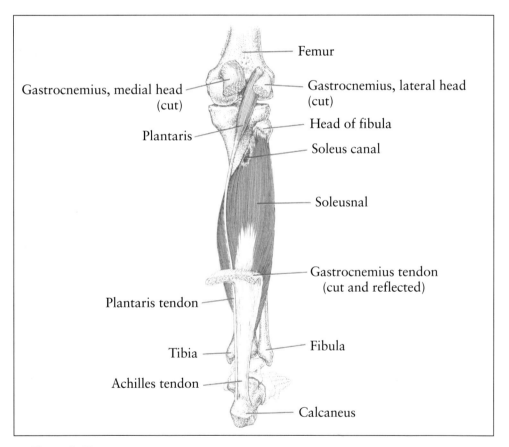

Figure 3-17

Posterior Leg

Prone Position (DVD 3, 20:56)

Figures 3-18 a and b. Prone Work on the Calf in a Stretched Position

Slowly sink into the posterior leg compartment and snowplow tissue to create length and softening. Note manipulation of ankle with the left hand or with the therapist's knee to provide stretch to the calf muscles. Specific work for the Achilles tendon will be shown later.

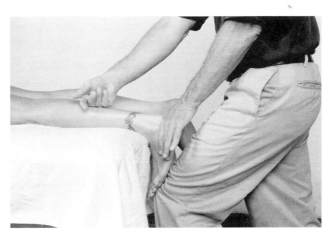

Figure 3-18a

Side-Lying and Supine Position

Figure 3-19. Side-Lying Calf Work

This strategy is effective for rolling the calf muscles away from the bone. Different amounts of stretch can be accomplished by flexing the ankle either passively or by having your client actively flex and extend the ankle.

Figure 3-20. Prone Calf Work to Stretch the Muscles

You may flex the ankle by pressing the ball of the foot with your axilla; this allows you to stretch

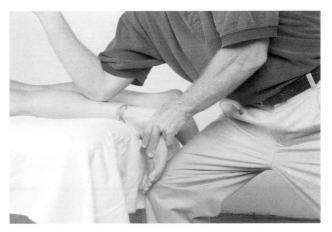

Figure 3-18b

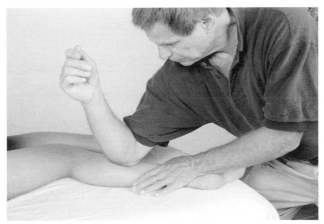

Figure 3-19

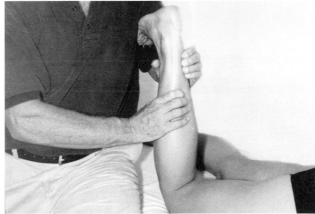

Figure 3-20

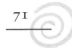

the posterior compartment. With very tight calves, stretching the calves while working may not initially be an effective way to sink into the tissue. It may be necessary to plantar flex the foot in order to soften the tissue so that your fingers can sink to a deeper level. After the muscles soften, you can then stretch the area and separate the two heads of the gastrocnemius muscle.

Figure 3-21. Anatomy of the Anterior Thigh and Pelvis

Notice the relationship of the quadriceps and the adductors, paying particular attention to the femoral nerve and artery, and to the circulatory structures as they descend through the inguinal triangle.

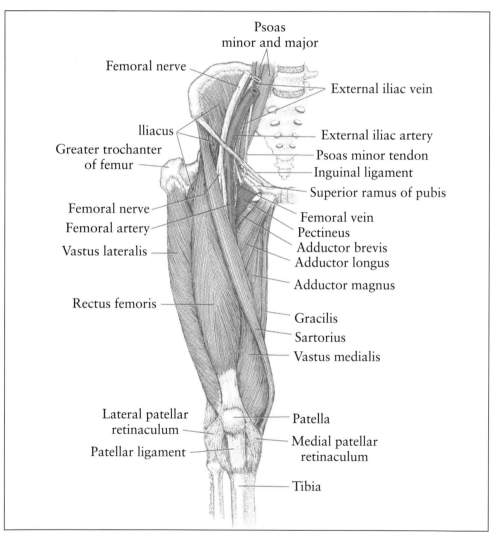

Figure 3-21

Figure 3-22. Anatomy of the Adductor Muscles

An awareness of the different angles of attachment of the adductors to the femur is necessary for precision in cross-fiber or longitudinal strokes and for separation of separate muscle compartments.

> *Origin: Lower pelvis and pubic bone*
> *Insertion: Medial femur*
> *Action: To adduct leg*

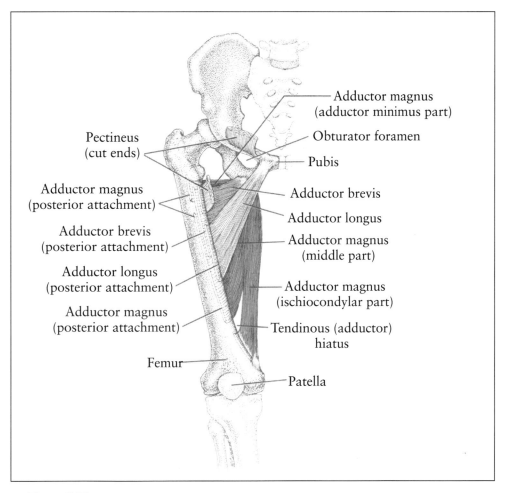

Figure 3-22

Figure 3-23. Anatomy of the Quadriceps Muscles

The rectus femoris is the only one of the quadriceps that crosses the hip joint, so it plays a major role in hip flexion as well as knee extension.

Origin: Trochanter of femur and anterior inferior spine of ilium

Insertion: Tibial tuberosity

Action: Knee extension

Hip flexion (only the rectus femoris)

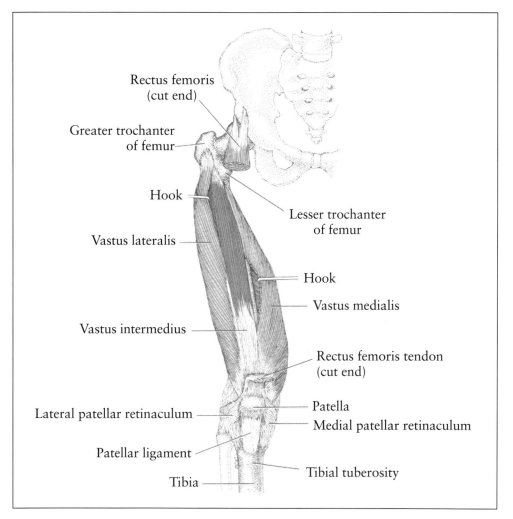

Figure 3-23

Figure 3-24. Anatomy of the Hamstring Muscles

All three hamstrings cross two joints and have the double function of hip extension and knee flexion. Because they attach at both the medial and lateral aspects of the knee, an individual muscle that is particularly tight can cause rotational stress upon the knee joint.

> *Origin: Ischial tuberosity and shaft of femur (for short head of biceps femoris)*
> *Insertion: Medial tibia (semimembranosus and semitendinosus) and fibula (biceps femoris)*
> *Action: Hip extension and knee flexion*

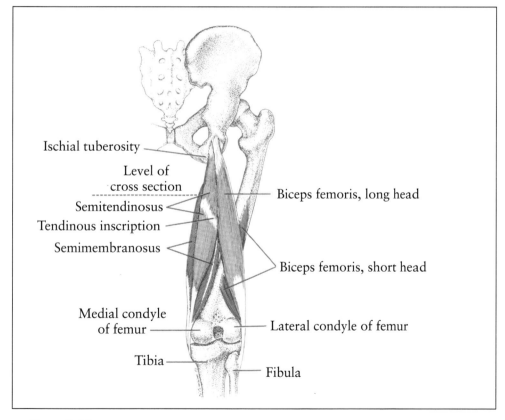

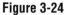

Figure 3-24

Working with the Upper Leg

Working the Adductors in Side-Lying Position (DVD 3, 1:01:20)

Tight and inflexible adductors can prevent the leg from swinging freely from the pelvis and can impose rotational stress on the entire leg and knee. Working on the medial leg in the side-lying position enables many options of leg placement to enable hip flexion or extension and knee flexion and extension. Broad lengthening strokes moving away from the pelvis are effective initially. After lengthening the adductors, precise separation of muscle compartments is effective in working with rotational forces exerted by the various adductors.

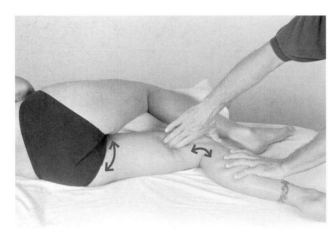

Figure 3-25

Figure 3-25. Side-Lying Adductor Work with Hip and Knee Positioning Options

Position the body comfortably and use a bolster to support the upper leg in order to minimize rotation in the back. Use forearm to lengthen tissue while extending knee with your other hand. To separate medial compartments, use fingers to define the different muscles. It is important to define the separation between the adductors and the quadriceps group, and also to define the separation between the adductors and the hamstrings. Arrows in this example show variations in knee flexion or hip flexion and extension.

Upper Leg Variations

Figure 3-26. Forearm Quadriceps Work

The forearm can be used to move proximally or distally. Be sure to exert oblique pressure and not to press directly into the bone. This technique is useful to work deep tightness, but is not precise enough to separate quadriceps compartments. Be sure to work slowly and not to compress the patella. Most forearm or elbow work will be in the direction of the muscle because there is not

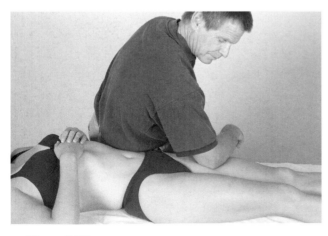

Figure 3-26

enough control of such long muscles for cross-fiber work in the belly of the muscle. In this case, the therapist is working away from the pelvis to decompress the hip joint. Use your other hand to internally or externally rotate the leg.

Figure 3-27. Supine Hamstring Work with Hip Flexion

This position offers the advantage of stretch to the hamstrings, which is not possible in the prone position. The entire length of the hamstrings can be worked in this position. The amount of knee and hip flexion is determined by the left hand and your shoulder height (stand to increase shoulder height). Try anchor and stretch techniques at the ischial tuberosity by anchoring the hamstring insertions with your knuckles or elbow and then flexing the hip joint.

Figure 3-28. Supine Hamstring Work with Knee Flexion and Extension Variations

Hamstring tightness is not limited to the belly of the muscle or the upper insertion. Many people are restricted behind the knee, and this limits full knee extension. Use the fingers to separate the heads of the hamstrings or gastrocnemius and stretch behind the knee. You may increase or decrease the amount of knee flexion (and therefore stretch) by either raising your own body, or by leaning backwards to extend the client's leg.

Figure 3-29. Ischial Tuberosity/Hamstring Insertion Work with Knuckles

Work anywhere on the hamstring with forearm, elbow, fist or fingers. Working the fibrous origin at the ischial tuberosity is often effective in relaxing the entire muscle group and will also relax the gluteals.

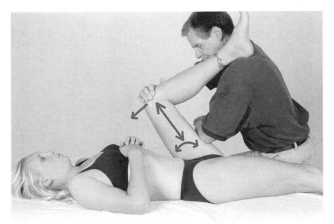

Figure 3-27

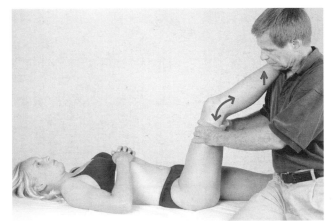

Figure 3-28

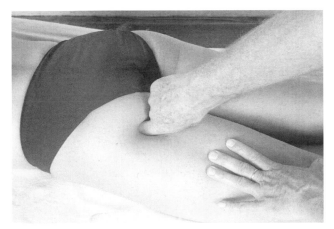

Figure 3-29

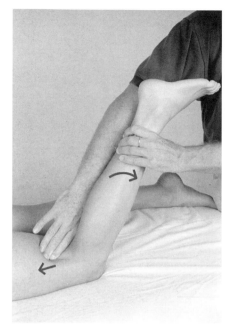

Figure 3-30

Figure 3-30. Posterior Knee Work (DVD 3, 49:19)

Flexing the knee softens posterior knee tissue, allowing for easier penetration to deeper layers. To localize stretch, try anchoring tissue with one hand while extending the knee. This is an extremely effective technique.

Abductors of the Leg

The lateral compartment of the upper leg also tends to be given perfunctory attention in a general massage. Attention to this area can offer great relief for a variety of complaints, including low back pain and knee pain. Be sure that any force is applied in an oblique direction rather than directly against the femur. Generally, work in a direction away from the acetabulum to decompress the hip joint. The forearm is an effective tool, but slow stretching work with the fingertips is also extremely effective and a better choice if the tissue is sensitive. Notice if the tissue is pulled posterior or anterior (which will cause rotational stress in the knee) and adjust the direction of your stretch accordingly.

Figure 3-31. Prone Abductor/IT Band Work

This method is most easily incorporated into a short massage when there is not enough time to do side-lying work. This position is contraindicated for clients with acute low back pain because of the rotational forces on the lumbar and sacral region and may also give some clients a feeling of sexual vulnerability. A pillow can provide cushioning below the inner thigh if needed.

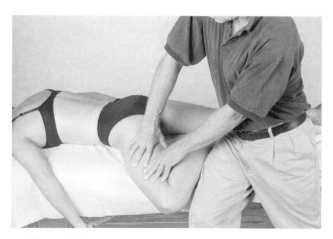

Figure 3-31

Figure 3-32. Supine Abductor Work

This is another nonspecific way of loosening the IT Band that is easily incorporated into a massage when you are not doing side-lying work. It is less threatening sexually than the prone position. For people with low back pain, it is also easier to minimize rotational forces on the lumbars, but still makes specific well-focused work difficult. It also can have a compressing effect upon the hip joint. Notice how the fist and forearm are stretching tissue in opposite directions.

Note: For less rotational stress on the back, place the foot on the near side of the opposite leg rather than across it.

Figure 3-33. Side-Lying Abductor Work (DVD 3, 1:02:25)

Of the three positions, this is the most versatile; the ability to bring the knee forward or back allows for many variations in the angle of the hip and knee flexion. Be sure to apply oblique pressure and to address the muscles above the hip joint, such as tensor fascia latae and the gluteals. If needed, a bolster will add support for the upper leg.

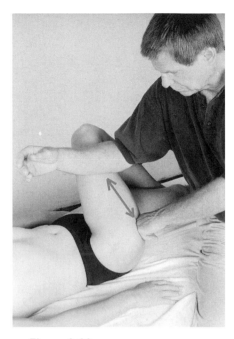

Figure 3-32

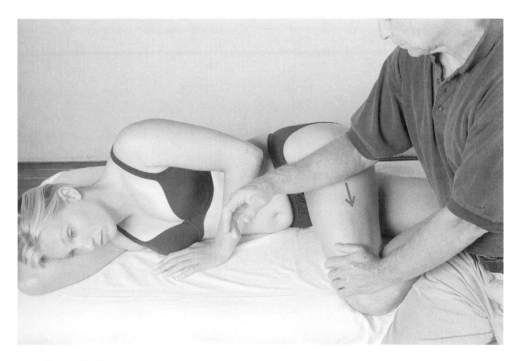

Figure 3-33

79

Tensor Fasciae Latae

Figure 3-34. Anatomy of the Tensor Fasciae Latae Muscle

The tensor fasciae latae is important to release the iliotibial band and normalize lateral strain on the knee.

Origin: Anterior superior iliac spine

Insertion: Iliotibial band

Action: Flexion, abduction and medial rotation of leg

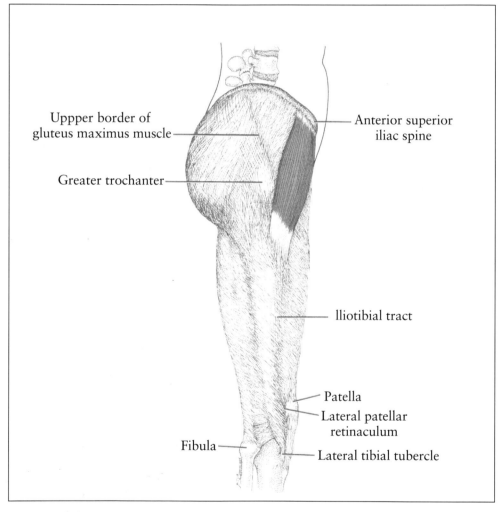

Figure 3-34

Figures 3-35 a and b. Defining the Borders of the Tensor Fasciae Latae Muscle

(DVD 3, 1:13:35)

Deep focused work with fingers, knuckles, or the elbow is more effective than broad strokes. Work the tendinous origin of the tensor fascia latae at the ilium, and notice if the muscle is rotated either forward or toward the rear, and work accordingly. Take care to differentiate and separate the anterior portion of the muscle from the quadriceps tendon and the posterior portion from the gluteals.

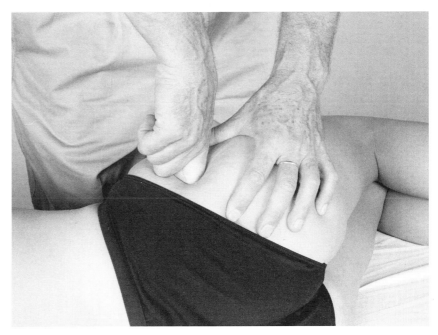

Figure 3-35a

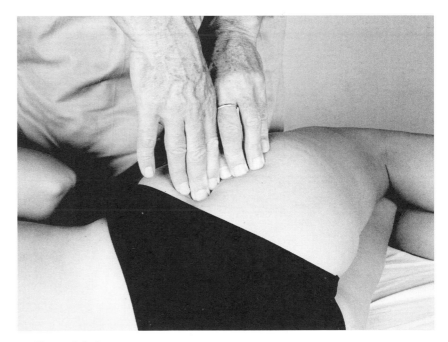

Figure 3-35b

Working with the Pelvis (DVD 3, 1:17:27)

Figure 3-36. Anatomy of the External Rotators of the Leg

Note the location of the sciatic nerve and the role of gluteus medius and gluteus minimus in abduction and maintenance of horizontality of the hip. The sacrotuberous ligament travels in a diagonal from the ischial tuberosity to connect with the sacrum beneath the gluteus maximus.

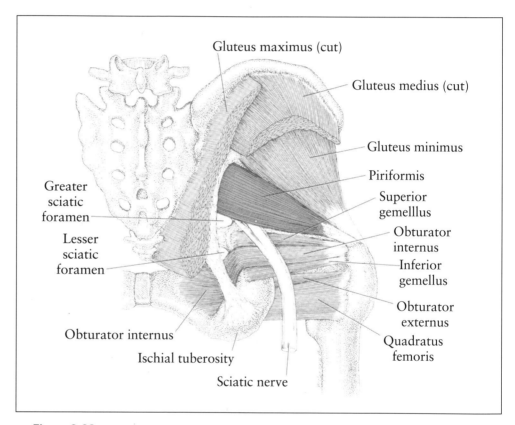

Figure 3-36

Gluteus Maximus Muscle (DVD 3, 1:26:40)

In order to access the deeper rotator muscles, it is necessary to soften and relax the gluteus maximus, which lies superficial to these muscles.

Figure 3-37. Working with the Gluteus Maximus Muscle

Work the medial border along the sacrum with cross-fiber strokes or with the intention of spreading tissue in a lateral direction. Longitudinal strokes with the fist, forearm, or elbow in a caudal direction are also effective.

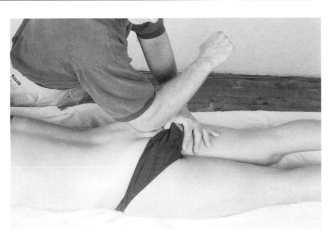

Figure 3-37

External Rotators of the Leg (DVD 3, 1:29:56)

The rotators are extremely important to address in clients who complain of low back tightness or sciatic pain. The sciatic nerve may be impinged by a tight piriformus muscle. The therapist needs to work *through* the external muscles such as the gluteus maximus. Using broad surfaces such as the forearm or fist makes it difficult to apply force with precision to the deeper muscles. If the therapist's fingers are strong enough, this is the best way to palpate and focus energy on the tight areas. The elbow will also work well. Often, just waiting with a steady pressure will effect a release. More specific directions for locating and treating the piriformis will be covered in Chapter Five.

Figure 3-38. Placing the Rotators in a Stretched Position

Positioning the femur so that the external rotators are stretched is a very effective technique. In this example, note that the knee is bent at a ninety degree angle to provide stability to the knee joint. Rotating the lower leg outward will act as a lever to internally rotate the femur and therefore place the rotator muscles in a stretch. The knee is stable if it is kept bent at a ninety-degree angle, but always check with your client to make sure that no strain is felt in the knee joint.

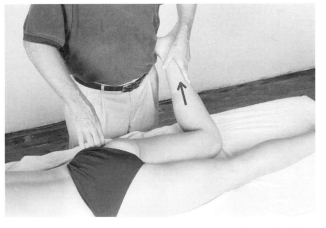

ⓔ Never press directly into the pelvic bones; always apply oblique pressure to guard against impinging the sciatic nerve that runs through this area. If the client has knee or hip joint problems, rotating the leg, as demonstrated, would be contraindicated.

Figure 3-38

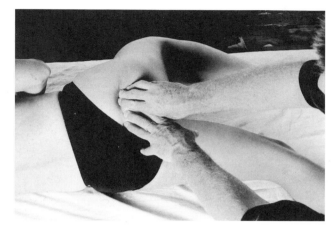

Figure 3-39

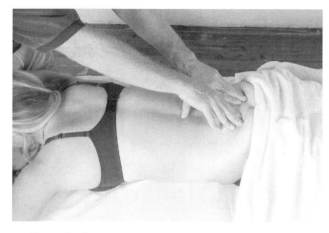

Figure 3-40

Figure 3-39. Side-Lying Work on the Piriformis Muscle

In the side-lying position, flexing the hip will stretch the piriformis muscle so you can work it.

Other Pelvic Options

The Sacrum (DVD 3, 1:23:31)

Working with the sacrum can have profound effects and calm the client very quickly. Superficial tightness of broad fascial tissue over the sacrum can disrupt the balance between the ilium and the sacrum and also affect lumbar function.

Figure 3-40. Spreading Tissue over the Sacrum

Take care to apply oblique pressure and never press straight down towards the table. Generally, tissue will be bunched medially, so gentle lateral spreading with the fingertips or knuckles will be effective and appreciated by the client. It is crucial to understand that you are not sliding over tissue or using much lubricant. This work is most effective if you master the concept of stretching tissue by anchoring with one hand and stretching in different directions away from this anchor. Work extremely slowly and patiently while waiting for tissue to melt or unwind from rotational patterns.

The Coccyx

Usually, one would not initiate work in this area unless the client requests it. However, since many clients will have experienced trauma to their coccyx at some time in their lives, it is useful to know how to work with it. The coccyx can be bent in an anterior angle approaching ninety degrees or may deviate left or right by several degrees. Careful palpation for fibrous build up unilaterally will indicate if work is needed.

Figure 3-41. Working with the Coccyx (DVD 3, 1:35:25)

Work through the towel or sheet that you are using as a drape. If you feel abnormalities in the coccyx, it is important to get permission from the client to work there. Work on the far side of the coccyx so that the soft pads of your fingers are in contact instead of your fingernails. Gently sink into the tissue on one side of the coccyx at a time. Initially, softening tissue is all that is suggested. If the client reports relief from pain or other benefits, work may progress in subsequent visits to gently attempting to straighten or return the coccyx to a normal position by applying very slow and gentle pressure while asking for feedback.

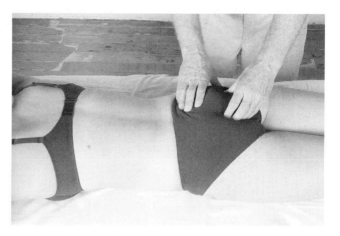

Figure 3-41

The Sacrotuberous Ligament

Different amounts of tension in each of the sacrotuberous ligaments (Figure 3-36) is often involved with sacral torsion problems. It can easily be envisioned that if one side is shortened and exerting more pull on one side of the sacrum, this rotational force may be manifested up the entire spine. The ligament is easily palpated by moving from the ischial tuberosity towards the bottom of the sacrum in a diagonal line.

Figure 3-42. Working with the Sacrotuberous Ligament

Longitudinal or cross-fiber strokes along the fiber with your fingers or knuckles are effective in softening the ligament. Depending on the amount of muscle or adipose tissue covering the area, sinking in with the point of the elbow and waiting for a "melt" is also effective. Remember that you are attempting to create balance between the two ligaments by softening the tighter side rather than working both sides equally.

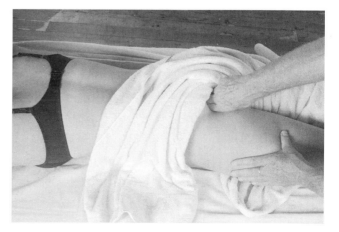

Figure 3-42

Working with the Pelvis and Low Back (DVD 4, 0:17)

Figure 3-43. Anatomy of the Iliolumbar Ligament and Quadratus Lumborum

Working with the iliolumbar ligament can be very effective in releasing low back tension and rotational stress. Because of the thickness of the lumbar fascia and muscles, it is necessary to use the fingers or knuckles instead of more broad tools in order to penetrate deeply enough.

> *Origin: Medial half of 12th rib*
>
> *Insertion: Posterior crest of ilium and iliolumbar ligament and to transverse processes of L4 and L5*
>
> *Action: Side-bending of lumbar spine (unilateral contraction) Lumbar extension and standing stabilization (bilateral contraction)*

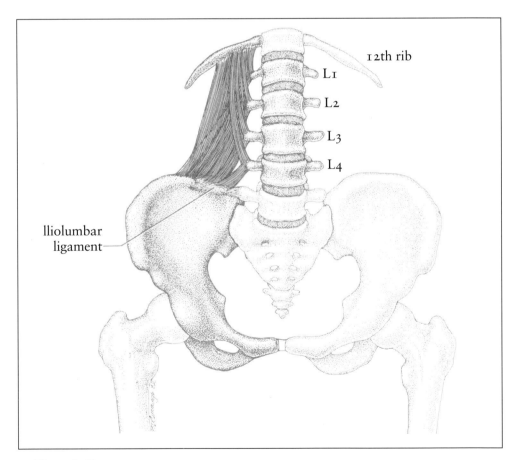

Figure 3-43

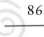

Quadratus Lumborum

Figure 3-44. Anatomy of the Quadratus Lumborum

The quadratus is more complex than is often shown in its attachment to the ribs and the crisscrossing of its fibers. Patient and precise work is necessary to effect release of these muscles.

Figure 3-45. Effect of the Quadratus Lumborum on Side-Bending

Quadratus muscles on the opposite sides of the spine may have very different tone and resting lengths. It is necessary first to compare the tension of both sides to determine a strategy to balance the two sides.

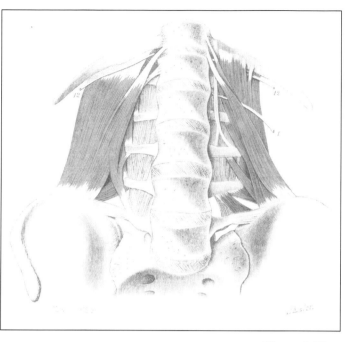

Figure 1-10

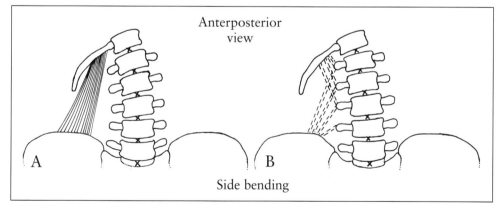

Anterposterior view

A   B

Side bending

Figure 3-45

The quadratus is an extremely important muscle that is often overlooked in general massage. If it is tight unilaterally, it can cause side-bending and spinal rotational problems (note that fibers insert on the transverse processes of L4 and L5 and could place unilateral rotational strain in this area). In the prone position, the quadratus is difficult to access and may require so much force to penetrate vertically that it is possible to disrupt the balance between the sacrum and the lumbar vertebrae. For this reason, it is best to access the quad-

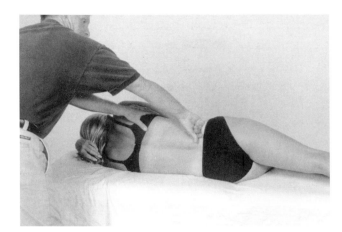

Figure 3-46

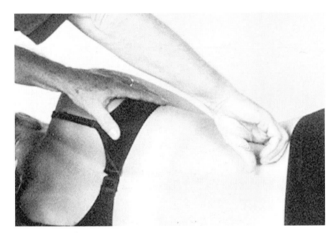

Figure 3-47

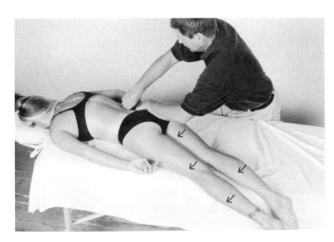

Figure 3-48

ratus in the side-lying position; this enables the therapist to position the legs in such a way that the muscle may be easily accessed and placed in various degrees of stretch.

Figure 3-46. Fist Work with the Quadratus Lumborum Muscle (DVD 4, 4:30)

To open the area, have the client side-lying with the top leg extended posterior and reaching down. The bottom leg should be bent forward to provide stability and minimize rotational forces on the spine. Work the insertions of the quadratus lumborum at its attachments at the 12th rib and at the crest of the ilium. The belly of the muscle can be worked both longitudinally and with cross-fiber strokes. If there is a noticeable difference in tightness from side to side, work the short side last. The crest can be worked with a broad surface such as the fist or forearm, but above this area, fingers allow the most precise work with the least disruption to surrounding tissue. Having the client's arm extended above the head will extend the ribs into an open position facilitating a greater stretch.

Figure 3-47. Knuckle Work with the Quadratus Lumborum Muscle

Using the fingers or knuckles will provide more precise and deeper access to the quadratus.

Figure 3-48. Stretching the Quadratus Lumborum in Prone Position

If it is inappropriate to work in side-lying position, and you wish to stretch the area, moving the feet to the opposite side of the table will stretch the quadratus and open the area for more easy access.

◎ Caution: Take care to not apply deep force over the kidneys. Also be aware that the floating ribs cannot tolerate too much pressure. If the muscle is extremely tight, it may be necessary to access it in a nonstretched position. It may take several sessions in order to relax the muscle enough to place it in a stretched position.

Working with the Abdomen

Figure 3-49. Anatomy of the Psoas Major and Iliacus Muscles

Notice how the iliacus and psoas muscles join to become the iliopsoas muscle.

Origin: Transverse processes and bodies of T-12 and lumbar vertebrae, intervertebral discs.
Insertion: Lesser trochanter of femur
Action: Lumbar extension when standing, lumbar flexion when bent forward, and (primarily) hip flexion.

Psoas and Iliacus Muscles

These two muscles combine to become the iliopsoas, but although they insert together on the lesser trochanter of the femur, each can be associated with different symptoms. Since the psoas originates from the lumbar vertebrae, it is more associated with spinal rotation patterns (unilateral tightness) and excessive lumbar curve or lordosis (bilateral tightness). Notice that the psoas also attaches to the intervertebral discs and could possibly be a factor in symptoms involving compression of discs. Since the iliacus attaches medially to the sacrum, tightness of this muscle has

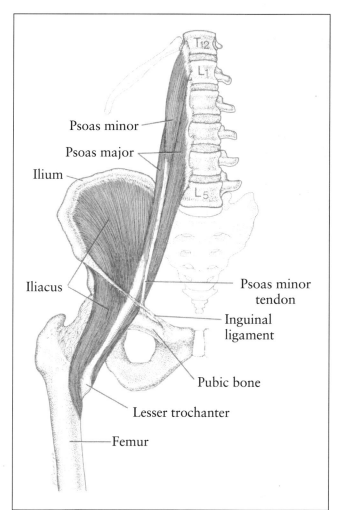

Figure 3-49

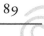

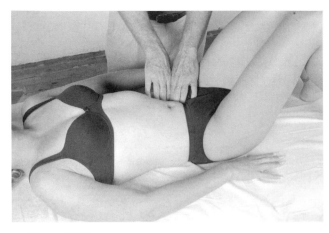

Figure 3-50a

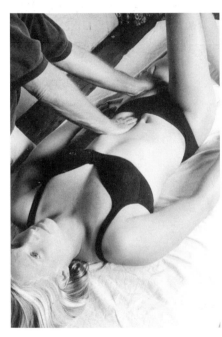

Figure 3-50b

more of a disruptive effect on the sacrum. Both muscles require patient and slow work that is not suited to an hour full-body massage. Explaining the anatomy of the muscles is often helpful for the client to understand discomfort she may feel in having treatment to this area.

Figure 3-50. Working with the Psoas Muscle (DVD 4, 24:14)

The client should lie in supine position with both knees bent comfortably. This position shortens and relaxes the psoas so that your initial work in the area will not be too intense. Have your fingers as soft as possible and slowly *sink through superficial tissue. Approaching lateral to the rectus abdominis at an oblique angle is often the easiest method of contacting the psoas. Have your hands at a slight diagonal, above but at a similar angle to a line drawn from the anterior spine of the ilium to the pubis. This will enable you to find the psoas without probing to determine if it deviates from the norm in its lateral/medial position.*

After palpating to determine if one side is shorter or tighter than the other, begin working unilaterally. Have the client slowly raise her foot to give both of you a clear sensation of the muscle. When the foot is being raised, determine if the muscle is tracking straight and is contracting properly rather than just allowing the other superficial hip flexors do most of the work. Longitudinal strokes at the level of the top of the pelvis and slightly caudal are usually the most effective. After you feel that some relaxation has been gained, allow the client to lower the leg on the side you are working in order to stretch the muscle. Continue your work on the iliopsoas in the leg extended position.

◎ Caution: Working on the psoas and anywhere in the inguinal triangle requires palpatory certainty (see Caveats section). Proper technique is extremely difficult to learn without supervision. If you have not had instruction in this area, either take a class or arrange a tutorial with an experienced teacher.

Figure 3-51. Bilateral Psoas Balancing

Bilateral psoas tightness can certainly be disruptive, but having only one tight psoas can be even more of a problem. This condition can place excessive torsion on the pelvis and spine as the tight psoas exerts rotational and side-bending force on the spine and pelvis. After you are satisfied with working the psoas unilaterally to soften and stretch whichever iliopsoas is tighter, it is useful to work bilaterally to give balance to the pelvis. Besides softening the muscle, part of your job may be to teach the client to use an underworked psoas by calling her attention to when one side is not contracting adequately.

This work may be done through the drape or towel. Sink in with your fingers bilaterally, a couple of inches above the inguinal ligament and have the client tuck the pelvis under similar to a subtle pelvic tilt. If one psoas jumps in an anterior direction or to one side, hold it as closely as possible in a neutral position.

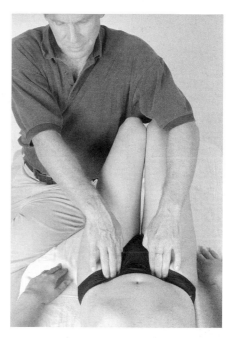

Figure 3-51

Figure 3-52 a and b. Working with the Iliacus Muscle (DVD 4, 36:30)

The iliacus muscles can also affect the rotational pattern of the pelvis. They are often associated with ilea that are pulled too narrow at the anterior superior iliac spine and need to open to a wider position. Because it attaches to the border of the sacrum, a tight iliacus muscle may be associated with sacral torsion.

With soft fingers, work the muscle along the inside rim of the pelvic bowl from either side of your client's body, waiting for the muscle to soften.

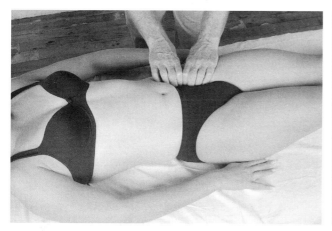

Figure 3-52a

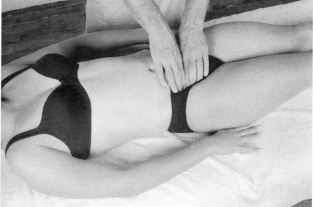

Figure 3-52b

◎ Precautions: Work in the pelvic area is contraindicated for women who have even the slightest possibility of being pregnant. Some women are also too sensitive to receive this work during their menstrual periods. Superficial fascia and muscle fibers in this area often run in one direction and are quite thin. Be cautious not to separate these fibers, which could cause a hernia. When working near the inguinal ligament, be aware of the femoral artery. You will be able to feel the pulse if you are near this artery. (See Caveats section.)

Working with the Breath (DVD 4, 17:20)

WHEN WORKING WITH THE BREATH, it is important to take the client's breathing patterns into consideration before planning a strategy. Pay particular attention to whether the client is *inspiration-fixed* or *expiration-fixed* and work accordingly.

Figure 3-53. Inspiration-Fixed Breathing Pattern (4, 13:39)
Inspiration-fixed breathers are often very tight in the low thoracic area of the back, and their anterior ribs are pulled up in front so that viewed from the side, their rib cages appear to be tilted upwards. From the front, the ribs and diaphragm of people with inspiration-fixed breathing patterns should be worked in a downward direction to let the front of the rib cage fall. Softening posterior muscles in the lower thoracic area will also help return the thorax to a more level position.

Figure 3-54. Expiration-Fixed Breathing Pattern (4, 14:43)
Expiration-fixed breathers usually need more work below the diaphragm in an upward direction and in the abdominal area to lengthen the rectus abdominis muscle.

Teaching a client to *belly breathe* as opposed to thoracic breathing is very helpful to ease strain to overworked scalenes and shoulder muscles which are working too

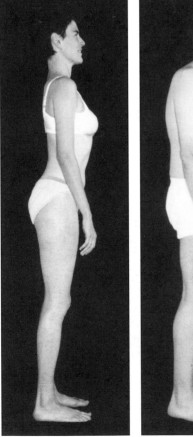

Figure 3-53   **Figure 3-54**

hard to lift the ribs. However, make certain that your instructions to breathe to the belly are not misinterpreted. Some new students of abdominal breathing overemphasize the new pattern and lose the ability of the chest to expand. Not only should the belly expand on the in-breath, but the breath should then continue up past the costal arch, and the ribs should expand also.

Working with the diaphragm can help make it possible for clients to take full breaths. It is important to open the area with preparatory work on the chest and abdominal muscles, and having the client bend the knees will soften the abdominal area for easier accessibility. Work slowly; have a dialogue with the client and don't be afraid to separate from clients to give them time to recognize and adjust to the changes in breathing patterns for several minutes.

Consider taking a workshop in breathing to increase your effectiveness in coaching in proper breath.

Figure 3-55. Grabbing the Ribs

Gently grabbing the lower ribs to stretch the rib cage will open the chest and diaphragm. Expedite the stretch by gently pulling the arm upward.

Figure 3-56. Releasing the Diaphragm

Often tissue is tight and immobile beneath the rib cage. This can pull the ribs down and impede breathing. Gently slide the soft part of your fingers under the ribs. Pushing tissue in that direction with your other hand will often allow for easier access. Do not force tissue to soften; this takes patience and needs to be a cooperative effort between you and your client.

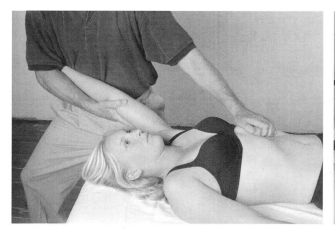

Figure 3-55

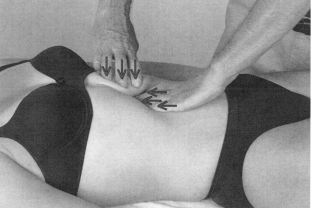

Figure 3-56

⊚ Caution: Take particular care on the right side of your client because of the location of the liver beneath the costal arch.

Many people only have the capacity to move the ribs in the front plane of the body so that you will be unable to feel significant movement of the ribs where they connect to the spine. Help the client connect his or her back to front so that the ribs appear to widen from the midline of the body in an anterior and posterior direction.

Aiding your client to breathe can be a great gift. Giving them a sense of breathing to the back as well as the front can be accomplished by holding your hands in front and back at the same time, having the client imagine spreading your hands with each breath.

Figure 3-57. Teaching an Awareness of Front-to-Back Breath Balance

Giving the client a perception of the connection between the front of the body and the back is very useful. Clients often report a whole new concept of breath as they gain an understanding of the interplay between the anterior and posterior planes of the body.

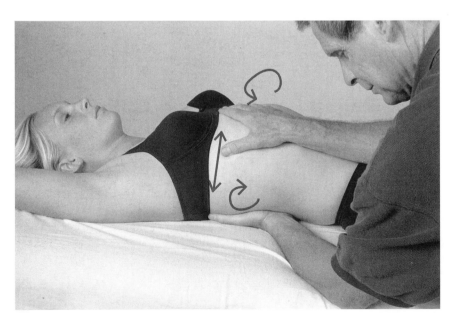

Technique 1: Have the client breathe to expand the ribcage in both anterior and posterior directions paying particular attention to softening the muscles of the posterior spine.

Technique 2: Do gentle "unwinding" by letting the hands move in a circular direction, sometimes in opposition to each other. (Taking a workshop in unwinding techniques is strongly recommended.)

Figure 3-57

Working with the Upper and Mid-Back (DVD 4, 45:41)

T HE PRONE POSITION IS THE MOST COMMON POSITION to approach the whole back. In this position, the lumbar fascia and muscles, the latissimus dorsi, erectors, lower and upper trapezius, and rhomboids are all easily accessed. These may all be worked with everything from fingers to elbows. Use of the forearms and elbows will cover the most area with the least amount of effort by using the therapist's own weight to apply force. Using fists and hands may require more muscular effort if the table is high. If using these tools, working farther away from the client with the arms extended makes possible using the legs and deep energy sources.

One problem with the prone position is that the muscles remain in a neutral position and (except by moving the arms above the head to manipulate the shoulder girdle) are difficult to place in a stretched position. For this reason, placing the client in side-lying position is an effective method of both stretching the muscles of the back and focusing forces to help mobilize the bony components of the spine. Use of pillows or other bolsters can help to maintain stability of the client. Variations in placement of the arms and legs offer many alternatives of rotation and stretch.

Figure 3-58. Distracting the Pelvis and Spine with the Forearm

Notice that the left elbow is next to the spine for more precise focus of force. If the right arm were used for the same stroke, it would not be possible to work with precision adjacent to the vertebrae. Working on the far side of the spine would require leaning too far forward so that the therapist's back would be stressed.

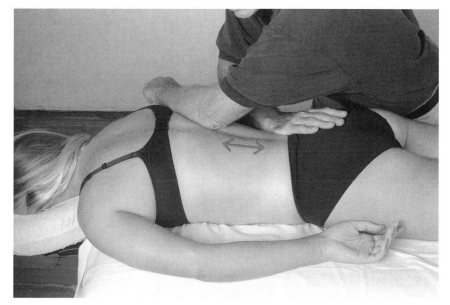

Figure 3-58

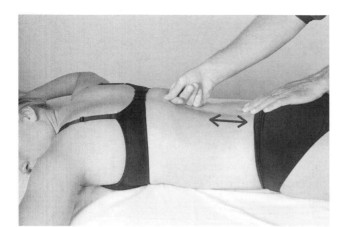

Figure 3-59. Distracting the Pelvis and Spine with the Fist

Both here and in Figure 3-58 the right hand is tractioning the pelvis in the opposite direction.

Figure 3-59

Vertebrae, Ribs, and Paraspinal Muscles

A quick examination of anatomy drawings of the paraspinal muscles demonstrates the intricate complexity of the intrinsic muscles that control small movements of the vertebrae. It is often these small, deep muscles that are responsible for the common back pain complaints of clients. However, many new students only focus on tight muscles and have never been taught to work with the vertebrae and ribs. And yet, it is essential for the therapist to direct attention to the mobility of the osseous components of the spine in addition to the muscular and soft tissue components. Providing mobility to vertebrae and ribs will often enable the adjacent muscles that are in spasm to relax. This can be accomplished by focusing rotational, anterior/posterior, and other mobilizing efforts to individual vertebrae rather than larger segments of the spine. Experimenting with varying degrees of flexion/extension and rotation when positioning the body will also aid in freeing vertebral fixations. Imagine the ribs as the keys of a piano; pay attention to the ease with which you can depress each of the "keys" with vertical pressure and how they are able to move up or down with the breath. See if you can notice areas of restriction or immobility.

When working on a client, after massaging the large external muscles so that they soften enough to allow penetration to deeper layers, it is useful to work slowly in the spinal groove between the spinous and transverse processes. It takes very little time to move down the spine and feel where vertebrae and ribs seem immobile. Gently rocking the vertebra from side to side by alternating pressure on each transverse process, gliding each vertebra forward, and testing rib mobility close to the spine will usually isolate several spots that require focused and precise work. Sometimes it is even possible to find a rib that is rotated so that instead of feeling a broad surface, it is possible to palpate the edge of the rotated rib. Gentle mobilization by slow rotation, both into and against the rotational pattern, or depression of the rib or vertebra will sometimes enable a profound release. Remember that ribs must be accessed lateral to the transverse processes. Such work is particularly helpful in areas where muscles refuse to soften regardless of how much attention they receive.

 Precise instructions for mobilizing vertebrae are far too complex to be discussed in this manual. Learning to work in this manner, however, is very possible for massage therapists. If you have an interest in learning these skills, an excellent book entitled *Spinal Manipulation Made Simple,* by Jeffrey Maitland, is available through North Atlantic Books.

Figure 3-60. Anatomy of the Paraspinal Muscles

Notice the importance of working in the area between the spinous processes and the transverse processes, or spinal groove. These deep and short muscles are often the cause of back pain rather than the large superficial muscles. Take your time to assess specific tightness with short strokes instead of always performing long flowing strokes to large muscle groups.

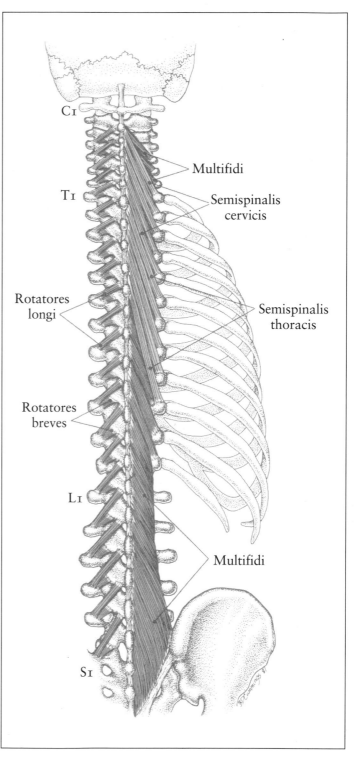

Figure 3-60

Figure 3-61. Anatomy of the Latissimus Dorsi Muscle

The latissimus dorsi exerts a profound effect upon the sacrum and pelvis, the lumbar and lower thoracic spine, and the ribs. Notice its action of internally rotating the humerus, making tension there a likely suspect in causing shoulders to rotate internally.

Origin: Lower six thoracic vertebrae, crest of ilium, sacrum, and lower four ribs

Insertion: Humerus

Action: Extends arm, adducts and internally rotates arm, depresses arm

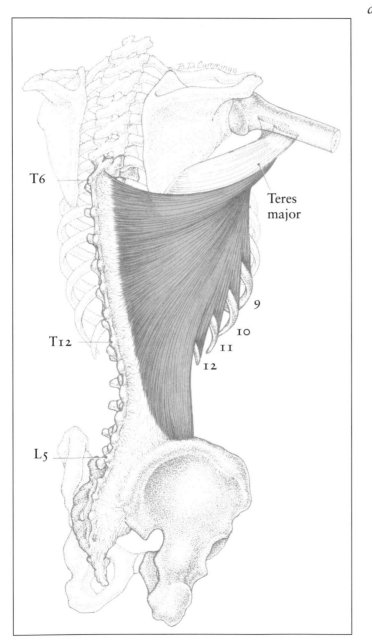

Figure 3-61

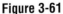

Figure 3-62. Anatomy of the Serratus Anterior

Notice the posterior attachments along the medial border of the scapula: a tight serratus anterior may account for tightly depressed scapulae, preventing access below the medial border.

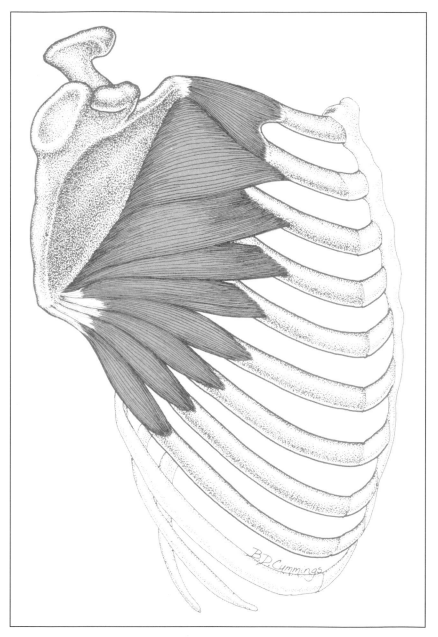

Figure 3-61

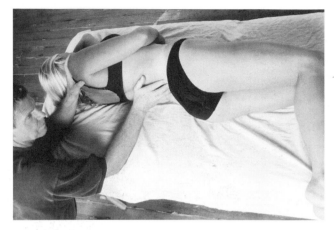

Figure 3-63

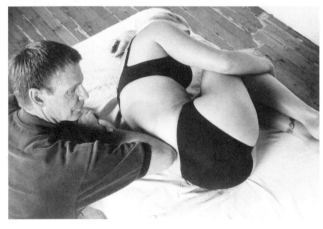

Figure 3-64

Side-Lying Techniques (DVD 4, 1:36:53)

Back Extension (DVD 4, 1:41:26)

Figure 3-63. Increasing the Ability for Low Back Extension \

Place the client's knees together and pull the feet back until you notice the lumbars being pulled forward. Work within your client's comfort range. As you achieve more flexibility, you will be able to pull the feet farther back. Reasons for treating the back in extension will be covered in Chapter Six.

Back Flexion (DVD 4, 1:37:44)

Figure 3-64. Increasing Low Back Flexion

Placing the client in a C-curve or fetal position allows for all of the major back muscles to be lengthened when working. This is a very comfortable posture for many clients regardless of whether they have particular back symptoms. This position is also very helpful for clients who have a pattern of too much lumbar extension ("sway back") because of tight lumbar fascia. Tucking the pelvis under lengthens this area and gives them the cue to let the pelvis drop naturally from the back rather than tightening the abdominal muscles to tuck the pelvis under. Have your client breathe and expand the ribs where you are applying force, or have her actively tuck her pelvis under to further lengthen the spine.

Work with the forearm or elbow is most effective for the broad muscles. Work in the spinal groove with fingers and knuckles is also very effective for the short paraspinal muscles; follow the spine all the way to the cervicals very slowly and stop to do repeat strokes in areas that are tight. Note that the "window wiper" (Figure 3-65) allows a great deal of leverage with minimal muscular force. The therapist should take care to bend his or her knees and protect the low back by keeping proper lumbar curve rather than bending forward from the waist.

Figure 3-65. Window Wiper Stroke

To add stability for broad strokes on the back, you can anchor your hand on the table and rotate your forearm back and forth similar to the wiper blades on an automobile. Be careful to not exert too much pressure or strain on your wrist; keep wrist flexion to a minimum. The distance at which you place your hand from your client's back will determine how sharp or broad the stroke will be.

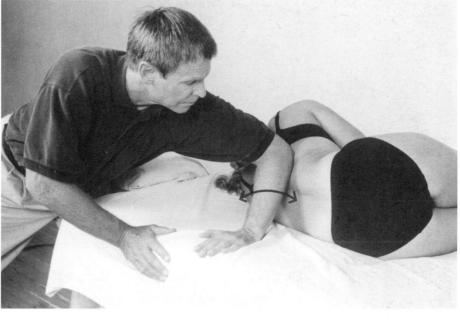

Figure 3-65

Spinal Rotation Techniques (DVD 4, 1:44:43)

These techniques are extremely helpful in increasing rotational flexibility, but should be applied with incremental increases to determine the tolerance of the client. They are contraindicated for clients with acute back pain; always err toward under-rotating rather than risking increased symptoms by exaggerating twist. The basic principle is to have the pelvis rotating in the opposite direction from the shoulder girdle in order to rotate the spine.

Figure 3-66. Opposing Pelvic and Shoulder Girdle Rotation for Spinal Mobilization

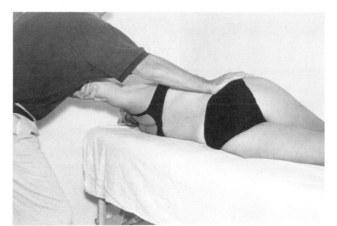

In this example, the right side of the pelvis is rotated forward by placing the top leg forward and drawing the bottom leg back. The shoulder girdle is rotated in the opposite direction by pulling the top arm back. Strokes can be long and broad, or more precise pressure may be applied by fingers or knuckles at specific areas where rotation is impaired as shown in the following figure.

Figure 3-66

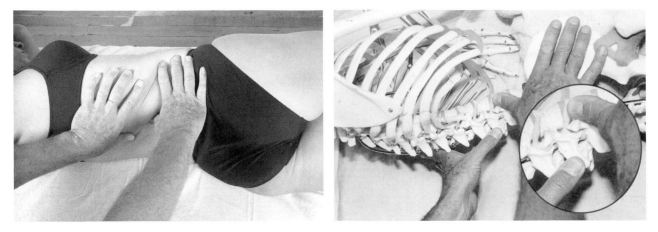

Figure 3-67a   **Figure 3-67b**

Figures 3-67 a and b. Spinal Rotation to Mobilize Vertebrae (DVD 4, 1:04:49)

These two photographs demonstrate techniques to create more rotational ability in the spine. When you notice that certain segments are inflexible, it is crucial to apply precise force to free movement where it is impaired. A broad, general stroke will free the spine where it is already flexible without mobilizing areas where vertebrae are immobile.

Focus your attention on the junction between two immobile vertebrae rather than on muscular tightness. Applying slow steady pressure, push the transverse process of the lower vertebra in an anterior direction. At the same time, push or pull the transverse process of the adjacent, upper vertebra in the opposite direction.

ⓒ To master these principles, it is crucial to have a clear understanding of how vertebrae articulate. In what plane do their facets articulate? It will be ineffectual to attempt to force vertebrae to move in directions or planes in which they are unable to move. Take the time to carefully examine a skeleton and notice the differences between the manner in which the facets of the cervical, thoracic, and lumbar vertebrae articulate. Spending a few minutes to conceptualize and understand how each group moves will open entirely new ways of working with the back.

For example, notice in the previous photographs that if you were to attempt to rotate the two vertebrae each in a manner opposite than shown, you would be pushing their facets together instead of opening the space to allow movement.

The rotation imposed by the twisted side-lying position will aid in the release. It may take a minute or more of patient pressure for the vertebrae to soften as the "stuck" facets become free moving again. Have your client breathe to the area and experiment with slight variations in flexion and extension to facilitate relaxation.

Figures 3-68 a and b. Spinal Rotation in the Opposite Direction

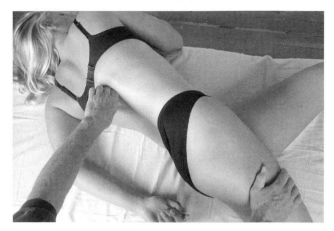

Figure 3-68a

To rotate the pelvis and shoulder girdle in the opposite direction from the previous example, simply reverse the position of both girdles. In this example, have the top leg pulled back and the bottom leg forward with the knee bent. The top arm is now pulled forward to rotate the shoulder girdle in the opposite direction. To increase the stretch, have the client's left arm behind the back in order to rotate the upper back into the opposite rotation. Although the photograph may appear somewhat contorted, this position is actually very comfortable. Remove any pillows from under the client's head to minimize cervical strain.

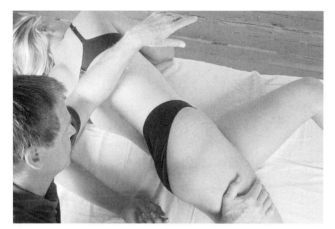

Figure 3-68b

Repeat both of these positions to the opposite side to create balance.

Working with the Shoulder Girdle and Chest

The shoulder girdle can be intimidating with its numerous muscles crisscrossing each other and having slightly different functions. Although there are exceptions, some general rules can greatly simplify working with the area. In most cases, the muscles concerned with internal rotation of the arm are located on the anterior surface of the shoulder, while external rotators are posterior. A great many complaints of shoulder joint pain are related to short and inflexible muscles that compress the shoulder joint. Relaxing any muscles that have a tendency to pull the humerus into the glenoid fossa will often decrease symptoms.

Many painful situations are due to protective holding of the joint. Gentle movement, especially with the joint distracted by slight traction, can override the protective shortening of muscles. Proprioceptive Neuromuscular Facilitation (PNF) stretches are particularly effective, but care must be taken to not overstretch and cause an increase in symptoms. PNF stretches are extremely effective for releasing tension and increasing mobility (see examples in Chapter Five), but the procedure is too complex to be taught in a manual. The basics are relatively easy to learn; it is highly recommended to take a workshop that teaches the skill.

Tightness in the upper chest will pull the shoulders forward and create strain in the upper back muscles that are attempting to counteract this tightness (see discussion on primary versus secondary shortness, in Chapter Six).

For this reason, it is important to give proper attention to the pectoralis muscles and chest fascia to create an opening of the chest. Otherwise, much of the attention to the thoracic spine will be wasted, if when the client finishes the massage, the back muscles have to contract again to counteract tightness in the anterior body.

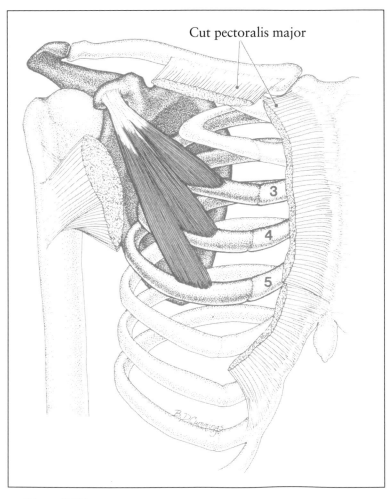
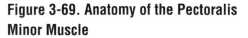

Cut pectoralis major

Figure 3-69. Anatomy of the Pectoralis Minor Muscle

The pectoralis minor attaches to the coracoid process of the scapula, and if it is short, can pull the shoulder forward.

Figure 3-69

Figure 3-70. Anatomy of the Pectoralis Major Muscle (Stretched)

This drawing, when compared with the next, illustrates how abducting the humerus is useful to stretch the pectoralis major.

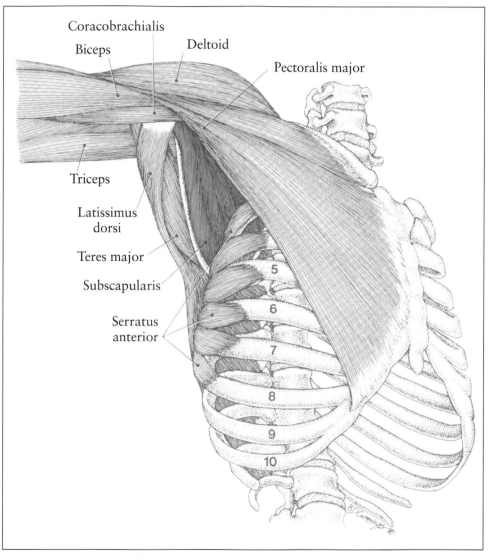

Figure 3-70

Figure 3-71. Anatomy of the Pectoralis Major Muscle

Notice the two origins of the pectoralis major and their different roles in adducting the humerus and internally rotating the arm.

Origin: Clavicle, sternum, and costal cartilage of 6th, 7th, and 8th ribs

Insertion: Humerus

Action: Adduction (and movement of arm across chest), internal rotation of humerus

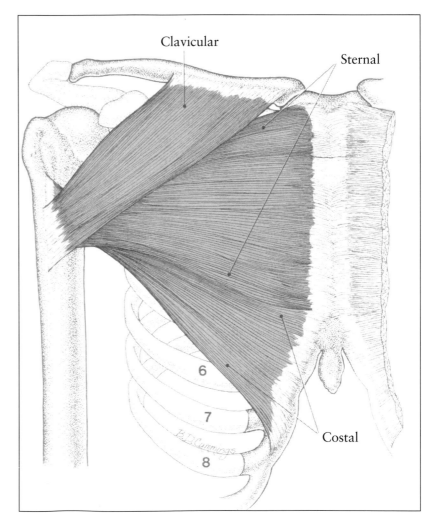

Figure 3-71

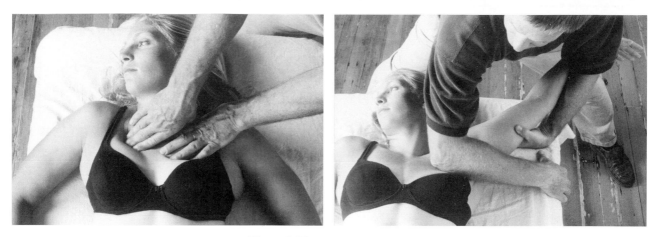

Figure 3-72   Figure 3-73

The Chest (DVD 5, 24:11)

In addition to specific work with individual muscles, broad fascial release work and rib mobilization can be very powerful—particularly with work on areas of emotional holding.

Figure 3-72. Superficial Pectoralis Major and Chest Fascia Work

Keep the fingers soft and apply force obliquely at a thirty-degree angle or less. Consider which direction you would like the tissue to release. Some clients will have their rib cages pulled down into a slumped posture, while others will have a more "military" posture and need to let their ribs fall.

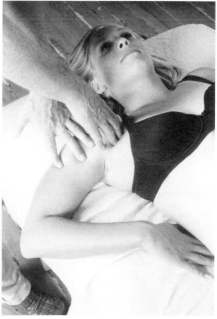

Figure 3-73. Stretching the Pectoralis Major

Broad strokes to the pectoralis major with fist or forearm are effective, especially if the therapist moves the client's arm to add stretch. Work this muscle at the sternum and at its insertion on the humerus. After initial softening has occurred, externally rotate the humerus by raising the arm above head in a comfortable position.

Figure 3-74. Pectoralis Minor Work

This muscle can be very sensitive. It must be addressed through the pectoralis major and is difficult to palpate. Working its insertion on the coracoid process is effective with the humerus internally rotated by pulling the elbow away from the body and in an upward position.

Figure 3-74

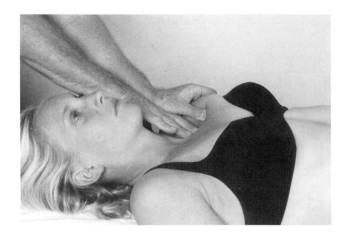

Figure 3-75

Figure 3-75. Differentiating the Pectoralis Major and Deltoid Muscles

In addition to kneading work, lifting the pectoral muscles or anterior deltoid from surrounding tissue will clarify the separation between muscle compartments and allow for more fluid movement of the arm.

⊚ Precautions: When performing deep work around the upper chest region, ask the client to inform you if they experience any nerve sensations. The thoracic outlet may be restricted and influenced by work that is actually fairly far removed from its exit. Also be cautious of the biceps tendon where it crosses the shoulder joint. It is vulnerable to inflammation from too aggressive work.

Figure 3-76. Anatomy of the Posterior Shoulder Muscles

Understanding the complex weave of the shoulder muscles requires a knowledge of the individual muscles and their specific actions upon shoulder movement.

Supraspinatus

Infraspinatus

Teres minor

Triceps (long head cut)

Teres major

Latissimus dorsi (cut)

B.D.Cummings

Figure 3-76

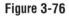

Figure 3-77. Anatomy of the Supraspinatus Muscle

Relaxing this muscle will help clients with compressed shoulder joints.
Origin: Supraspinatus fossa of scapula
Insertion: Greater tubercle of humerus
Action: Abducts arm and pulls head of humerus towards
glenoid fossa

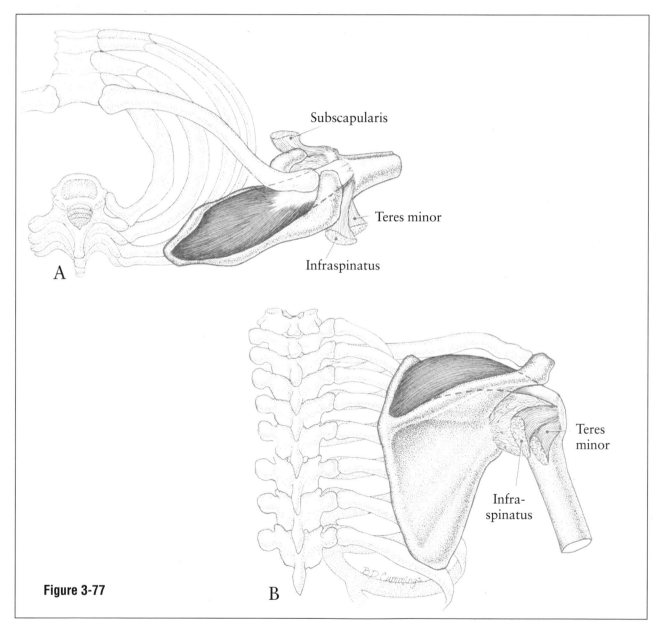

Figure 3-77

Figure 3-78. Anatomy of the Infraspinatus Muscle

Because of the angle of pull of the lower fibers of the infraspinatus muscle it is an important muscle for depressing the humerus in the glenoid fossa so that the joint is not impinged when raising the arm.

Origin: Infraspinatus fossa of scapula

Insertion: Posterior aspect of greater tubercle of humerus

Action: Externally rotates arm and depresses humerus when raising arm

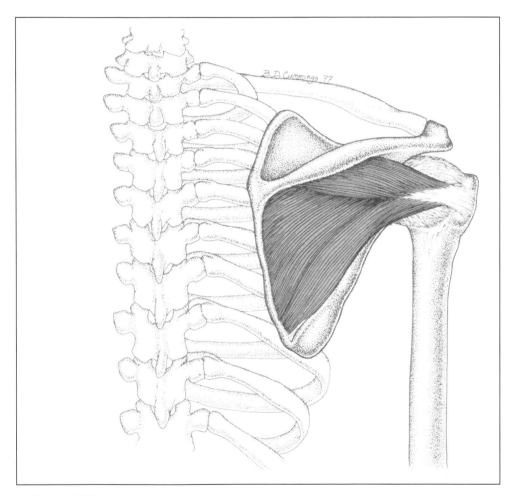

Figure 3-78

Figure 3-79. Anatomy of the Teres Major Muscle

To distinguish its action from the teres minor, it is important to note that the teres major is an internal rotator of the arm.

> *Origin: Lateral dorsal scapula*
> *Insertion: Merges with latissimus dorsi to anterior aspect of humerus*
> *Action: Internal rotation and aids in resisted adduction of arm*

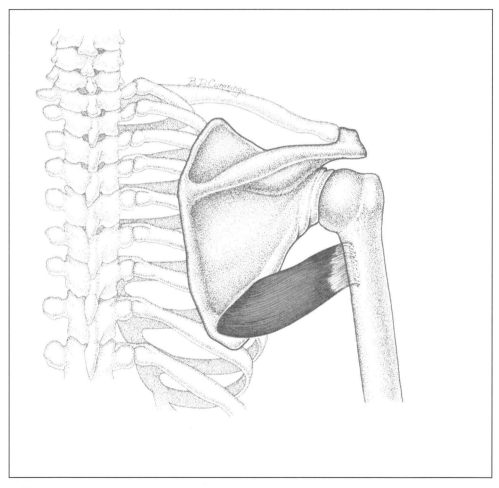

Figure 3-79

Figure 3-80. Anatomy of the Teres Minor Muscle

The teres minor is an external rotator of the arm.
Origin: Dorsal surface of scapula near axillary border
Insertion: Posterior greater tubercle of humerus
Action: External rotation of arm and depression of humerus

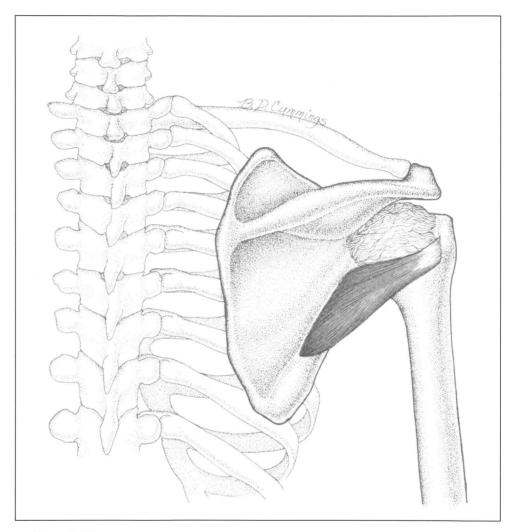

Figure 3-80

The difference in rotational action of the teres muscles is important for determining a working strategy. For an internally rotated humerus, the teres major would need lengthening, while an externally rotated humerus would need work on the teres minor.

Most of the rotator cuff muscles are susceptible to overuse injuries or traumatic injury in sports or activities involving a throwing motion. In addiction to their specific roles in rotation and other arm movement, they play an important role in decelerating the arm in a throwing motion because they are the antagonists of large muscles that are pulling the arm forward with great speed and force. Even if your client does not complain of pain, softening and lengthening the rotator cuff muscles will enable more fluid movement and help to prevent injuries, especially to athletes.

Figure 3-81. Anatomy of the Subscapularis Muscle

In addition to internally rotating the arm, the subscapularis acts to depress the humerus in the glenoid fossa, and with the arm in a fixed position can rotate the scapula.

> *Origin: Internal surface of*
> *scapula*
> *Insertion: Lesser tubercle of*
> *humerus*
> *Action: Internally rotates*
> *arm and stabilizes*
> *humerus in glenoid*
> *fossa against*
> *deltoid's action*

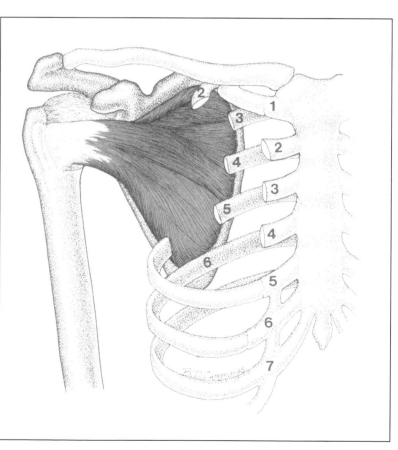

Figure 3-81

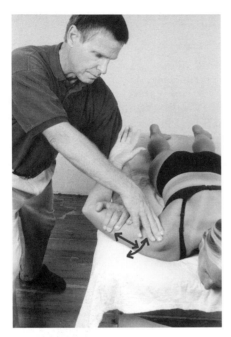

Figure 3-82

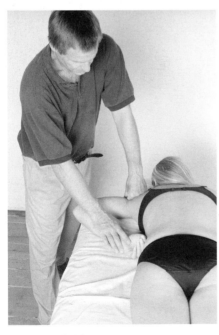

Figure 3-83

The Rotator Cuff (DVD 5, 0:23)

General relaxation of this area can be accomplished by broad strokes using the fist or forearm. Fingers or knuckles are useful to separate the compartments between the individual muscles. Usually these muscles will be too short and tight, which compresses the shoulder joint; placing the arm in a position to stretch the muscles will aid in release.

Figure 3-82. Manipulating the Arm to Work with the Rotator Cuff Muscles

For working on the right shoulder in prone position, grasp the humerus with the left hand. Placing your forearm under the client's forearm or wrist enables you to manipulate the arm into internal or external rotation, and at the same time abduct or adduct the arm and apply force to either distract or compress the joint.

Figure 3-83. Static Placement of the Arm to Stretch the Rotator Cuff Muscles (Prone Position)

With the client prone, abduct the elbow to stretch the area into internal rotation. With the arm in this position, both of your hands are free to perform meticulous work on the individual rotator cuff muscles.

The Scapula (DVD 5, 11:39)

The scapula is the "cam" upon which most of the upper thoracic and shoulder muscles exert their influence. It may elevate, lower, move medially or laterally, flare in or out, and rotate. Some people have scapulae that are bound on all sides so that they are immobile. Understanding which muscles are restricting movement is crucial to forming a strategy for freeing the area.

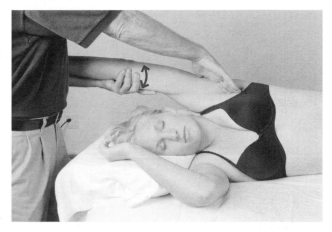

Figure 3-84

Freeing the Lateral Scapula

Figure 3-84. Side-Lying Technique for the Lateral Scapula with Fingers

Work with precision on the teres major and minor, subscapularis, and the latissimus dorsi to free the scapula from the ribs. Use your other hand to rotate the humerus and abduct the arm to focus stretch.

Figure 3-85. Side-Lying Lateral Scapula and Ribs with Forearm

This work is similar to the previous example but is less specific. The broad application of force by the forearm or elbow is better accommodated by ticklish clients. Focus on broad fascial sheets with less emphasis on specific attachments of muscles. This is particularly important for clients with "winged scapulae" which may be a result of tightness around the lateral scapula.

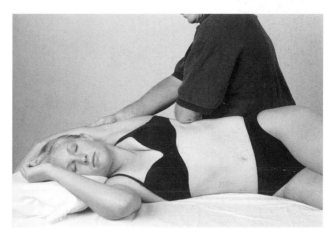

Figure 3-85

Figure 3-86. Side-Lying Lateral Scapula Rotation with Fingers

Grabbing the scapula and rotating or stretching it in other ways feels good and can increase mobility.

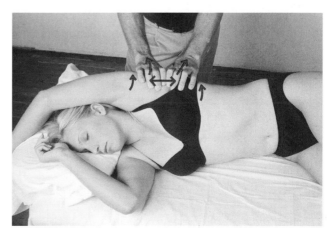

Figure 3-86

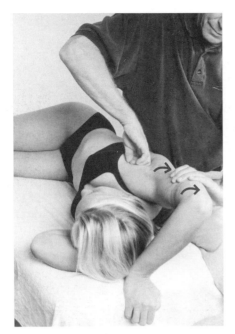

Figure 3-87

Figure 3-87. Side-Lying Lateral Scapula with Knuckles

Use of the knuckles is effective in releasing the scapula from the ribs.

Figure 3-88. Side-Lying Lateral Scapula with Elbow

The elbow is a very effective tool to save your fingers and knuckles for another day.

Figure 3-89. Supine Lateral Scapula with Fingers

It is not necessary to place your client in side-lying position to access the lateral scapula. While working with the fingers or knuckles, manipulate the client's arm to place the lateral muscles in a stretch. If the area is very tight or sensitive, then lowering the arm a small amount will soften tissue and make the area more accessible.

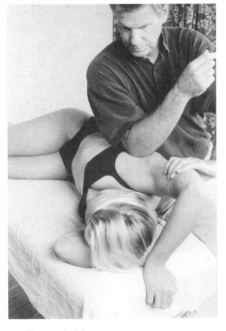

Figure 3-88

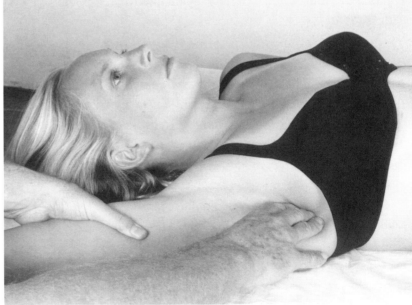

Figure 3-89

Freeing the Medial Border of the Scapula
Figure 3-90. Freeing the Medial Border of the Scapula (DVD 5, 9:51)

Brace your right arm with the elbow on the table while pulling the shoulder back with your other arm. This will give access to the medial scapula and the subscapularis muscle.

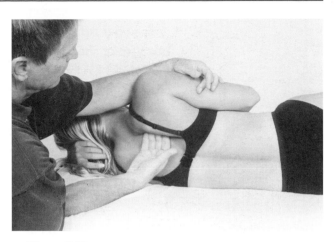

Figure 3-90

Figure 3-91. Distracting and Rotating the Scapula

Once you have the scapula in hand, you may pull it away from the body and manipulate it in any number of ways from elevation, to rotation, to distraction.

Working with the Arms (DVD 5, 37:15)

◎ If I were to send a "Recall Notice" to all of my earlier clients based upon what I now know, I would have them come back for all of the work I neglected to give to their arms. It is not surprising that massage therapists often pay only perfunctory attention to the arms. Except for athletic injuries and some serious overuse or repetitive strain syndromes, most clients rarely complain about arm tension. Although the arms may not often be a source of pain, their holding patterns transmit stress past the shoulder girdle all the way through the neck to the cranium. Begin to notice how people hold their arms. Do they hold their elbows out, pull

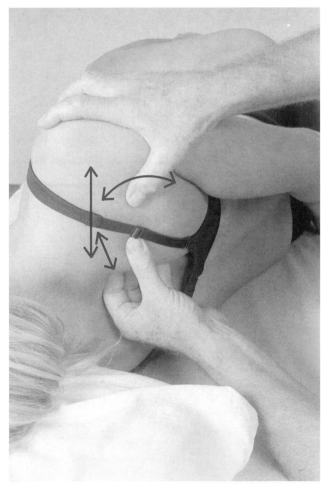

Figure 3-91

their upper arms back with their triceps, have too sharp an angle at the elbow because of short biceps? Do their arms, elbows, and wrists swing freely when they walk? Do their thumbs or do the backs of their hands face forward? I have had countless clients comment that their shoulders and neck feel completely different after focused work to release arm tension. Have a fellow massage therapist work only on your arms for fifteen minutes or more and then stand up and notice how different your shoulders and neck feel.

Don't forget to work both the lower biceps and triceps to free the elbow joint. To experience the relationship between elbow holding patterns and shoulder tension, stand and tense your elbows. Notice how the strain travels to your shoulder and trapezius muscles; it is almost impossible to relax the trapezius muscle if your elbows are tight. In class, we demonstrate this relationship by picking someone with obvious elbow tension, working on just one arm, and then having the model stand to show how the shoulder on that side relaxes.

The use of fingers, knuckles, the fist, forearm, or elbow are all acceptable for work on the arms. Notice in the photographs that the therapist's other hand can manipulate the stretch on muscle groups by flexing or extending the elbow and wrist and also by pronating or supinating the forearm to work on either wrist flexors or extensors.

Figure 3-92. Supine Triceps Work

Abducting the arm above the client's head and varying the amount of bend in the elbow will stretch the triceps. Some clients will be unable to comfortably let their arm relax above the head; notice the use of a bolster to support the arm if this is the case. Be sure to move slowly so your client will know how you are moving her arm. It is not necessary to ask clients if they have had injuries to the shoulder; they will usually tell you as you begin to lift their arms, or you will be able to feel protective holding mechanisms. If your client has ever had a dislocated shoulder, be sure to keep the arm adducted to the side and refrain from externally rotating the humerus, especially if the arm is raised.

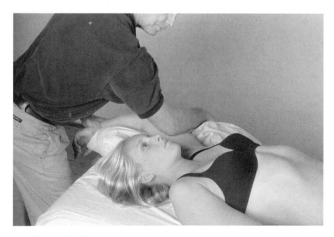

Figure 3-92

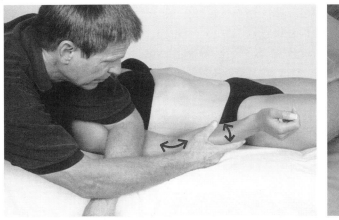

Figure 3-93

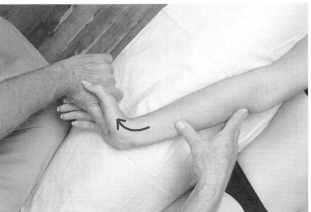

Figure 3-94

Figure 3-93. Biceps Muscles

For short biceps it is helpful to begin with the elbow flexed to soften the muscle for easy access. Work in the direction of muscle lengthening as you extend the elbow.

Figure 3-94. Wrist Flexors (DVD 5, 41:06)

Work the inside of the forearm while extending the wrist to stretch the wrist flexors. Instead of using your thumbs, the forearm or fist are effective tools.

Figure 3-95. Wrist Extensors

These muscles are often more fibrous than the wrist flexors and benefit from more precise work to separate compartments. Flex the wrist to place the wrist extensors into a stretched position.

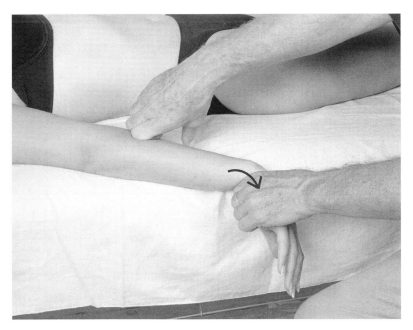

Figure 3-95

Working with the Hands (DVD 5, 46:05)

Figure 3-96. The Hands

The fingers, knuckles, and even the elbow are effective for working on the hands. Try not to use the thumbs for deep work here. The palm is rarely stretched into opening, so using the nonworking hand to spread and open your client's hand is very useful.

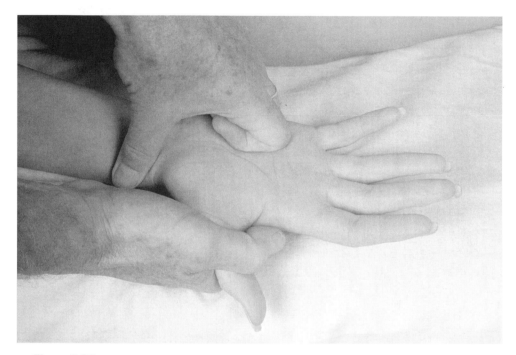

Figure 3-96

Working with the Neck (DVD 5, 49:47 through 1:08:32)

As common as complaints of neck pain are, how often have you had a client arrive complaining that it hurts to hold the neck in a neutral position while looking straight ahead? Such symptoms are rarely experienced. Except for a rare condition called torticollis, people complain of neck pain when they move their head and neck through certain ranges of motion. And yet, most of the neck work performed in a massage is done in the neutral (nonrestricted) position.

The vast majority of neck problems are due to the articulation at the facets of each vertebra with its adjacent neighbor. The ability of osteopaths and chiropractors to correct misaligned vertebrae explains their popularity. As massage therapists, we can not attempt to adjust vertebrae, but we can become extremely proficient at locating where vertebrae are not moving properly and softening spasmed muscles that are the potential cause of the immobility. If there is one skill that will ensure a thriving practice, knowing how to work with a neck in different positions to return normal function is that skill. The knowledge of how to work with the cervical vertebrae is a rewarding and fun pursuit that should continue to improve throughout your career as a massage therapist.

An examination of the following anatomical drawings demonstrates the complexity of the forces acting upon the cervical vertebrae. It also demonstrates why, as good as it may feel, broad, unspecific massage to the large superficial muscles of the neck and shoulders usually does not resolve complaints of neck pain and immobility. The small intervertebral muscles are usually the cause of pain and the stiff necks that our clients so often complain of.

It is not extremely important to know the names of the specific small muscles that control the intricate movements of the cervicals and of the skull's articulation with the atlas. It is crucial, however, to be able to palpate and work with these muscles through large superficial muscles such as the trapezius and levator scapulae in order to restore balance to the neck.

The key to working with the neck is to begin to focus on the relation of each vertebra to the adjacent vertebrae above and below it. How does it rotate, side bend, flex, and extend relative to its neighboring articulation? Which tiny muscles that connect these vertebrae are in spasm? How can you gently move the neck to place it in a neutral or pain-free position near its end range of movement so that you can effectively work? These skills take many years to develop, and like most of our knowledge of massage, are incremental in their acquisition. Strive to constantly learn more about the neck and how it works. Begin by palpating the transverse processes and determining areas of sensitivity. If you take the time to be able to locate areas of inflammation with precision, you are on your way. Slowly build on these early skills to cultivate your talents of palpation and techniques for working with the neck. Being able to treat the neck can be the bread and butter of a successful massage practice, and it will add fun and gratification to your work.

Figure 3-97. Anatomy of the Major Neck Muscles

The observation of the crisscrossing muscles of the neck with their various functions shows the importance of specific work rather than just broad superficial strokes to relax the neck. Try to determine if the neck is tighter in the anterior or posterior muscles, or if one side holds more tension.

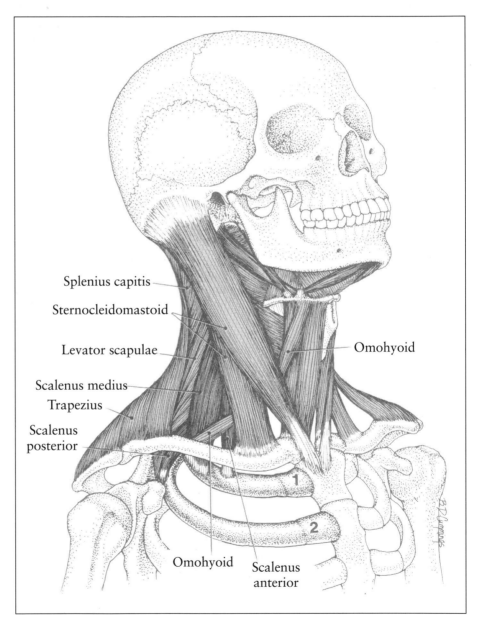

Splenius capitis

Sternocleidomastoid

Levator scapulae

Scalenus medius

Trapezius

Scalenus posterior

Omohyoid

Omohyoid

Scalenus anterior

1

2

Figure 3-97

Figure 3-98. Side-Lying Trapezius Techniques (DVD 5, 18:15)

It is important to relax the large superficial muscles to facilitate working on the smaller and deeper muscles. Placing your client into the side-lying position allows easy access to the trapezius muscle with the added advantage of allowing more stretch to the muscle. Either passively push the shoulder down, or better yet, ask your client to actively reach toward her feet.

Figure 3-99. Anatomy of the Layers of Cervical Muscles

There are sometimes six or seven layers of muscles covering the cervical spine. It is often necessary to budget your time to include time needed to soften the external muscles in order to contact the deeper muscles which control the intrinsic movement of the vertebrae.

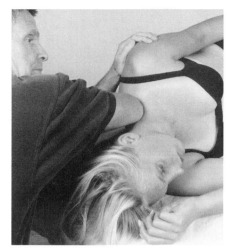

Figure 3-98

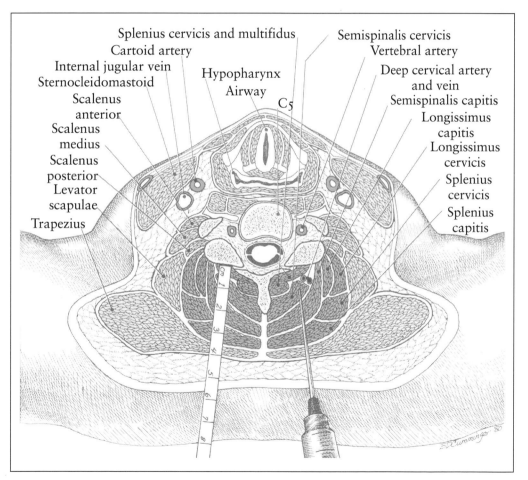

Splenius cervicis and multifidus
Cartoid artery
Internal jugular vein
Sternocleidomastoid
Scalenus anterior
Scalenus medius
Scalenus posterior
Levator scapulae
Trapezius

Hypopharynx
Airway
C5

Semispinalis cervicis
Vertebral artery
Deep cervical artery and vein
Semispinalis capitis
Longissimus capitis
Longissimus cervicis
Splenius cervicis
Splenius capitis

Figure 3-99

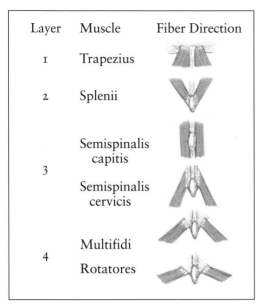

Layer	Muscle	Fiber Direction
1	Trapezius	
2	Splenii	
3	Semispinalis capitis	
	Semispinalis cervicis	
4	Multifidi	
	Rotatores	

Figure 3-100a

Figures 3-100 a, b, and c.
Anatomy of the Deep Cervical Muscles

When clients complain of neck pain when turning the head, it usually is the small muscles that travel from one vertebra to the next in diagonal directions to rotate the vertebrae. It is not necessary to know the names of these muscles, but it is crucial to be able to sink through superficial muscles to palpate particular individual muscles and effect their release.

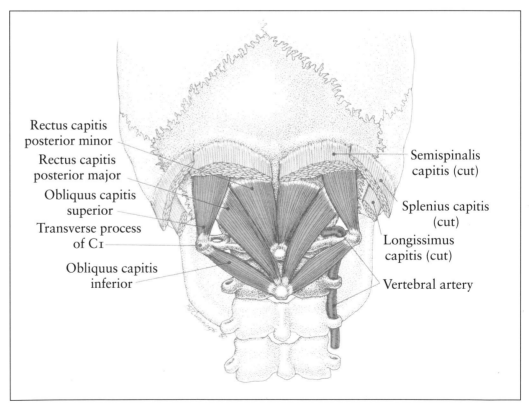

Rectus capitis posterior minor

Rectus capitis posterior major

Obliquus capitis superior

Transverse process of C1

Obliquus capitis inferior

Semispinalis capitis (cut)

Splenius capitis (cut)

Longissimus capitis (cut)

Vertebral artery

Figure 3-100b

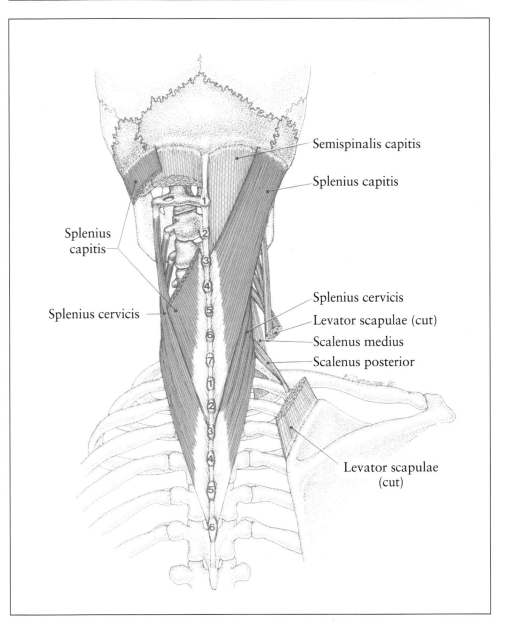

Semispinalis capitis

Splenius capitis

Splenius capitis

Splenius cervicis

Splenius cervicis

Levator scapulae (cut)

Scalenus medius

Scalenus posterior

Levator scapulae (cut)

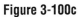

Figure 3-100c

The First Rib and Its Importance for Neck Work (DVD 5, 33:34)

Sometimes neck problems are actually the result of lack of mobility in the thoracic vertebrae and the ribs. The first rib is particularly vulnerable; it may be immobile, rotated, or pulled up and compressing nerves against the clavicle. The good news is that it is fairly easy to help restore balance to the first rib. The best way to learn is to have someone who is experienced work on your first rib so that you can know what it feels like. Many workshops that cover neck work automatically teach protocols for mobilizing ribs. Almost always, rib problems are a result of immobility rather than instability. They become slightly rotated or in some other way deviate from normal position, and the tissue at their articulations becomes hard and inflexible in an attempt to prevent further deviation. Particular ribs then become "stuck."

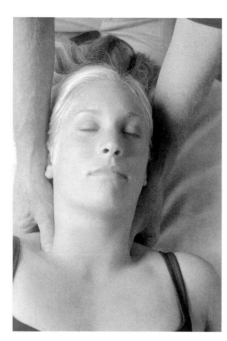

Figure 3-101

Figure 3-101. Mobilizing the First Rib

Palpate the first ribs with your thumbs immediately in front of the trapezius muscle. Notice if one rib is elevated more than the other, but most important, determine if one rib is more mobile than the other. Determine if a rib is rotated by feeling for a sharp edge rather than the flat surface you would expect with a normal rib position. Try to create balance in freedom of movement by applying steady pressure directly on the rib itself and waiting for tissue to soften and for a slight improvement in the mobility of the rib.

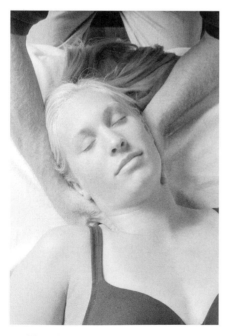

Figure 3-102

Figure 3-102. Side-Bending Mobilization of the First Rib

After determining which side needs more work, work unilaterally. Side-bend the client's head towards the side you are working and with your thumb, gently depress the head of the rib next to the transverse process of the first thoracic vertebra. Initially, a steady pressure will be all that is required, but if you do not feel movement, try side-bending your client's head slightly more and experiment with a slow, pulsating pressure. Do not try to force a rib into movement; work gently and slowly with small adjustments in neck rotation, flexion/extension, and side-bending.

Working with the Anterior Neck (DVD 5, 53:43)

Figure 3-103. Anatomy of the Scalenes Muscles

The scalenes are crucial to address in order to provide balance between the anterior neck muscles and the posterior muscles. People who are chest breathers overwork these muscles to elevate the ribs on inspiration. In some ways, these muscles could be compared to the iliopsoas muscles in their action on the spine. In the same way as the psoas pulls the lumbar spine forward into an exaggerated curve when the legs are fixed, the anterior and medial scalenes can pull the cervical vertebrae forward if the ribs are fixated in a low position. Conversely, if the neck is held erect by overworked posterior muscles, then short scalenes can pull the ribs up against the clavicles and compress the thoracic outlet.

ANTERIOR SCALENES

> *Action: A. Bilaterally: Neck flexion*
> *B. Unilaterally: Side-bending*
> *C. If neck is fixed, aids in respiration by raising first rib*
>
> *Inserts: A. Superior: Anterior tubercles of transverse processes of C-3 to C-6*
> *B. Inferior: First rib*

MEDIAL SCALENES

> *Action: Same as anterior scalenes*
> *Inserts: A. Superior: Posterior tubercles of transverse processes of C-2 to C-7*
> *B. Inferior: First rib*

POSTERIOR SCALENES

> *Action: Stabilizes neck in neutral position*
> *Inserts: A. Superior: Posterior tubercles of transverse process of C-6 and C-7*
> *B. Inferior: Second rib deep to levator scapulae muscle*

→

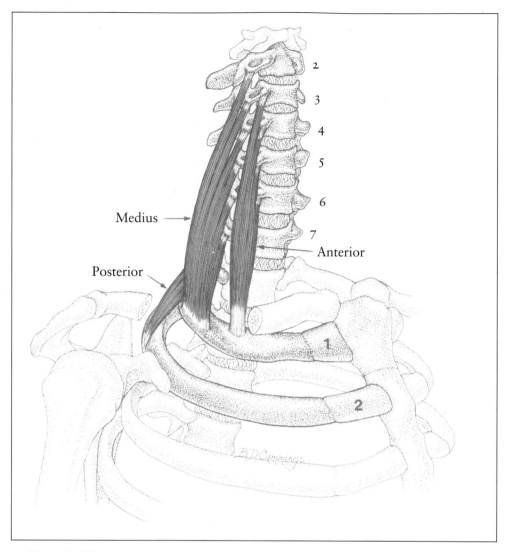

Figure 3-103

Figure 3-104. Working with the Anterior Scalene Muscles

These muscles insert behind the clavicular head of the sternocleidomastoid muscle. Work from the clavicle by initially elevating the client's head and then dropping it back while anchoring the sternal attachment and then working the belly of the muscle. When working unilaterally, have the client rotate and side-bend the head to the opposite side while anchoring the insertion. Stretch the skin to work under the clavicle on the first rib.

Generally work unilaterally, but initially palpate to determine if one side is tighter. Support the head with one hand in order to flex, extend, or rotate the cervicals. Flexing the neck forward enables access below the clavicle. Once you are anchored on tight aspects, extending the head posterior will stretch the muscle. Anchor anywhere you feel tightness and select the appropriate movement to stretch the area. Follow the anterior scalenes up to their attachment on the transverse processes of the cervical vertebrae.

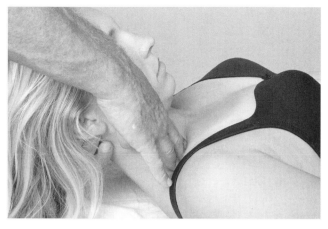

Figure 3-104

◎ Precautions: Because of the proximity of the thoracic outlet, ask your client to inform you of any nerve sensations down the arm. Also, be aware of the carotid pulse and do not work directly above the artery.

Figure 3-105. Working with the Medial Scalenes Muscles

Work in a manner similar to the way you worked with the anterior scalenes, or in side-lying with upper arm supported by the lower arm (as in Figure 3-106) to access the clavicle and first rib. Work lateral to clavicular head of the sternocleidomastoid muscle slightly posterior to the anterior scalenes. Remember to be cautious about the carotid pulse and any nerve sensations. Notice that turning your client's head will add stretch to the scalenes.

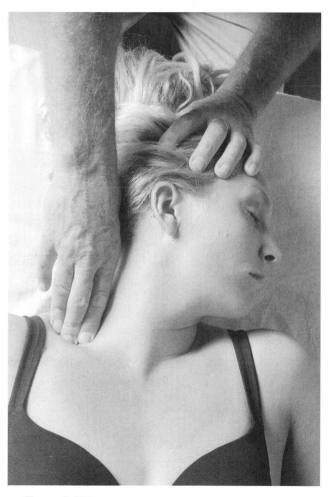

Figure 3-105

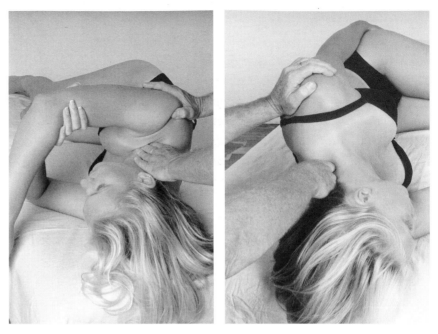

Figure 3-106　　　　　**Figure 3-107**

Figure 3-106. The Arm-Supported Side-Lying Position

Having your client support her upper arm allows the use of both of your hands. This position is effective in lifting the clavicle away from the ribs so that you can work on the scalenes insertions on the ribs.

Figure 3-107. Working with the Posterior Scalenes Muscles

Both prone and the side-lying position enable easy access to the area. See next section, which covers working the neck in the prone position.

ⓔ Many of the following strategies for neck work will suggest positions and rotations to mobilize vertebrae. Most important—never attempt to force a vertebra to move. Work gently and let movement occur rather than making it happen.

Strategies for Prone Neck Work (DVD 5, 49:53)

When working with your client in the prone position, a headrest is almost a necessity for comfort and to keep the neck in a neutral position for extended periods of time. However, the neutral position does not always inform you about restrictions to movement and problem areas. For this reason, it is often a good idea to have your client turn her head to each side to work on the neck to improve rotation and side-bending. It is much easier to rotate the head and neck if they are bent forward into flexion. If you have a tilting head rest, it is a simple procedure to flex the neck, but this option does not allow for much side-bending or rotation of the cervicals. Thus, it is often a better alternative to place a pillow under your client's chest so the head can drop comfortably forward, can rotate to either side, and can also side-bend. These options allow for many different combinations of cervical position, which will enable you to increase the range of movement in the neck. If your client has low back pain, you can also place a pillow under the stomach to decrease the lumbar lordosis caused by the pillow under the chest.

Figure 3-108. Freeing Tight Cervical Vertebrae in Prone Position

Visually examine the spine to determine if there are any specific areas where the rotation and side-bending are not smooth. Think small rather than globally; you are interested in individual vertebrae rather than large muscle groups. Palpate vertebrae for their ability to rotate and move in other planes. The palpation by itself will feel good to your client and will begin to free vertebrae. When you encounter tight paraspinal muscles, sink in with soft fingers and wait for softening. Never force vertebrae to move, but begin to free up "stuck" areas by rotating one vertebra in one direction while anchoring its neighbor so that movement is localized at a particular facet. As you gain practice, you will be able to intuitively move the neck into slightly different positions while you work, which will further increase your effectiveness at focusing rotation at individual areas of tightness.

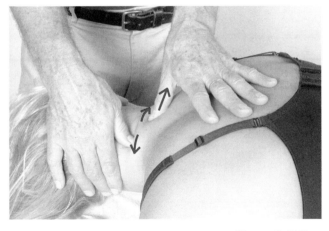

Figure 3-108

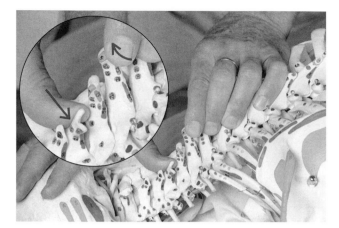

Figure 3-109

Figure 3-109. Demonstration of Technique with a Skeletal Model

Notice how you can use the processes of the vertebrae as small levers to aid in rotation.

Working with the Skull
(DVD 5, 1:08:39 through 1:17:04)

Figure 3-110. Anatomy of Some Cranial Muscles

Working the muscles and fascia of the skull is an important way to expand and solidify your work in the cervicals. The muscles of expression in the face often hold tension and respond well to lengthening strokes rather than strokes that just compress tissue with the goal of energetic relaxation.

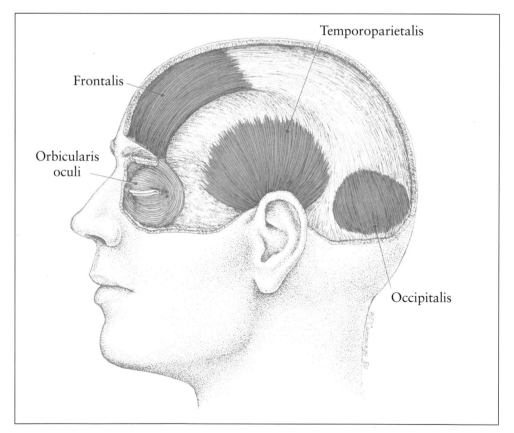

Figure 3-110

The Occipital Ridge

Figure 3-111. Working with the Occipital Ridge and the Mastoid Process

The occipital ridge from the mastoid process to the posterior midline is extremely important to treat. This will "finalize" much of the work performed on the bellies of all the inferior neck muscles that attach here and will also relax many of the superior skull muscles. If you are limited for time, two or three minutes of work here will accomplish as much as ten or more minutes of nonspecific work to the posterior neck muscles and will often relax deep muscles which are inaccessible with the superficial neck work because you will be addressing their tendons where they insert on the occiput.

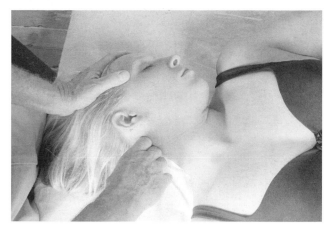

Figure 3-111

General Skull Work

Figure 3-112. Broad Fascial Work on the Skull

Nonspecific soft finger work to large areas of the skull feels good to the client and can dissipate scalp tension in a very short time. Gently stretch and unwind tight tissue over the temporal, occipital, and parietal bones. Remember not to work directly over the sphenoid area. Palpate localized tension areas approximately the size of a dime and apply slow, steady pressure until the area softens. Clients love this work. Be careful not to pull hair; remember that you are working with tight fascia and muscles beneath the skin. You should visualize *grabbing* this tissue *rather than sliding over the skin and hair.*

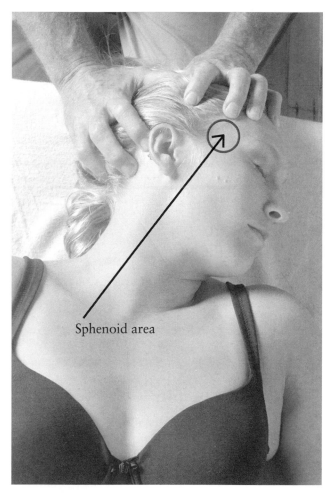

Sphenoid area

Figure 3-112

133

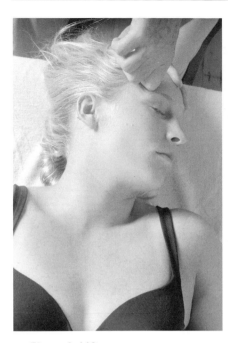

Figure 3-113

Anterior and Medial Skull Work

Figure 3-113. Working with the Forehead

Do not be afraid to use knuckles on the skull. The temporalis and frontalis muscles often hold a great deal of tension. Have the client open her mouth, frown, or even imagine emotional states that are often held in these areas to demonstrate the connection between feelings and localized tension.

Working with the Jaw and TMJ

Serious TMJ dysfunction is a complicated disorder, and it is not the role of a massage therapist to attempt to "fix" this condition. However, working with the external muscles can give relief to some clients, and sometimes enable long-term improvement. For permanent improvement, addressing the cause of the problem with changes in behavior of the client is usually the best approach. Education in proper chewing, jaw relaxation and strengthening exercises, proper posture and support for the cervicals during sleep all can be of benefit. Mouth braces to keep from grinding the teeth during sleep (bruxism), and elimination of harmful habits such as chewing gum often prove helpful.

Even if the client does not experience pain in the jaw and skull, relaxing external muscles associated with the jaw and creating balance between the left and right sides can have profound effects upon the client's relaxation. It is important only to attempt to create better balance and smooth opening and closing rather than striving to totally alleviate pain. Do not attempt to create too much change in one session. Often demonstrating to the client how much tension resides in this area by just relieving a small amount of strain will be greatly appreciated. For clients who have more serious problems, doing careful meticulous work may prove beneficial, but referring to specialists is advisable.

Figure 3-114. Anatomy of the Temporalis Muscle

Place the pads of your fingers over your temporal bone and bite down. You will feel the temporalis muscle contract. For many people, this muscle holds tension and can affect jaw function.

> *Action: Closes jaw*
> *Inserts: A. Above:*
>   *temporal bone,*
>   *frontal bone, zygo-*
>   *matic arch*
>   *B. Below: coronoid*
>   *process of*
>   *mandible*

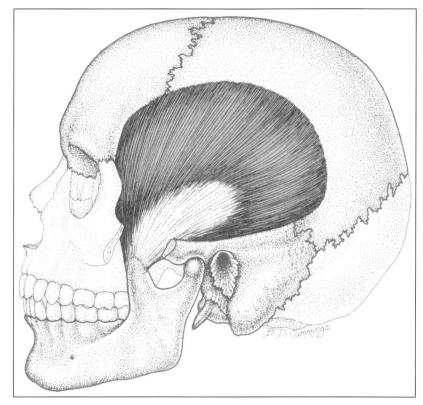

Figure 3-114

Figure 3-115. Working with the Temporalis Muscle

Any jaw work should include work with the temporalis muscle. Work the belly of the muscle for trigger points, and have your client open her jaw to demonstrate how the muscle stretches. Having your client bite down will also demonstrate the action of the muscle to teach self-massage. Also work the insertion of temporalis by opening mouth one-half inch to access the coronoid arch of the mandible.

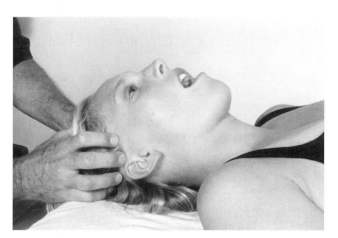

Figure 3-115

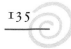

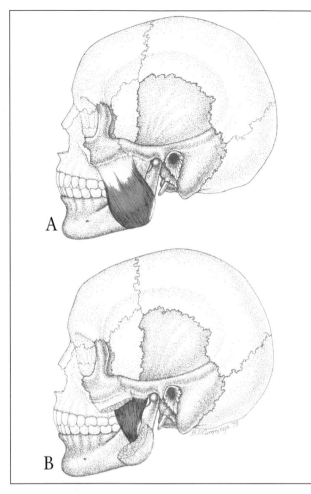

Figure 3-116

Figure 3-116. Anatomy of the Masseter Muscle

Palpate the masseter on yourself by biting down. Like the temporalis, this muscle is frequently tight and responds well to even short periods of massage.

   Action: Closes jaw

   Inserts: A. Superior: Zygomatic process of maxilla and zygomatic arch

   B. Inferior: External surface of mandible at its angle and inferior half of ramus.

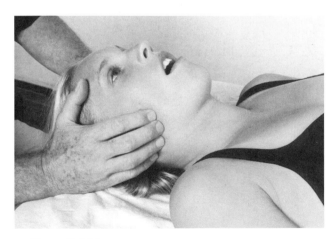

Figure 3-117

Figure 3-117. Working with the Masseter Muscle

Work cross-fiber and also in the direction of the muscle. Pay particular attention to origin and insertion. Work with mouth open to stretch muscle or closed to soften the muscle for easier access. Be certain that you are working on muscular tissue rather than salivary glands, which will be softer. If you have any doubt, ask your client to bite down so you can define the boundaries of the muscle.

Figure 3-118. Anatomy of the Lateral Pterygoid Muscle

The lateral pterygoid lies deep to the masseter and must be accessed by working through the masseter. Open the jaw one inch and work at its attachment at the condylar neck and ramus of the mandible.

> *Action: Closes jaw (lower portion)*
> *Aids in opening jaw (upper portion)*
> *Protrusion of mandible*
> *Lateral deviation of mandible to opposite side*
> *Inserts: A. Anterior: Sphenoid bone*
> *B. Neck and ramus of mandible*

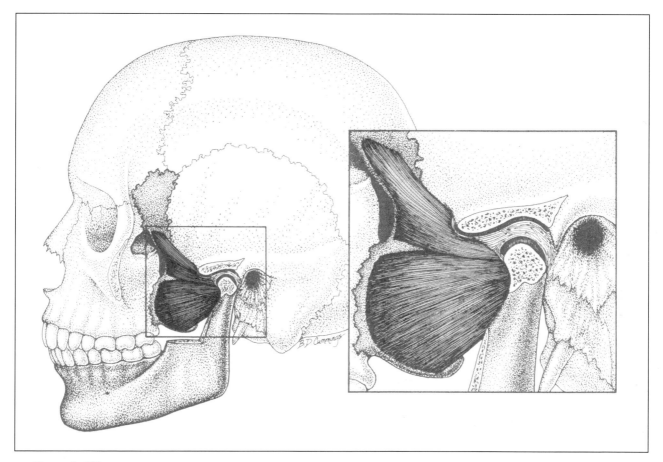

Figure 3-118

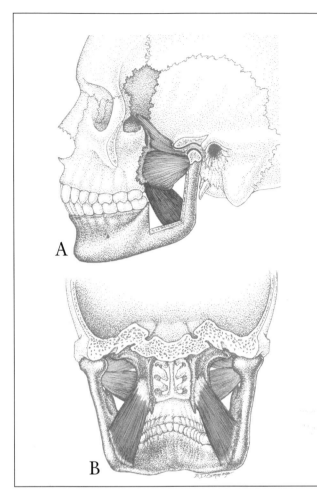

Figure 3-119

Figure 3-119. Anatomy of the Medial Pterygoid Muscle

This sling-like muscle is often a very important factor in jaw tension. It is best accessed by working inside the mouth using latex gloves. Inter-oral work is beyond the scope of this book, but if you are interested, take a workshop in treatment of jaw tension or TMJ. The following description demonstrates how to access the lower attachment of the medial pterygoid muscle.

    Action: Closes jaw

    Inserts: A. Superior: Medial surface of lateral pterygoid plate

              B. Inferior: Lower border of ramus of mandible, close to angle of jaw

Figure 3-120. Working with the Medial Pterygoid Muscle

Work the lower insertion on the inside of mandible. Have client clench jaw to palpate the insertion of the medial pterygoid as it tightens and then have her relax as you sink into the muscle with soft fingers.

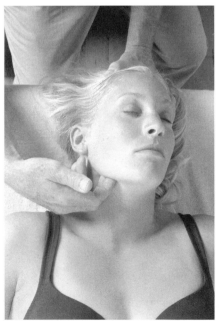

Figure 3-120

Figure 3-121. Anatomy of the Digastric Muscle

This interesting muscle moves the hyoid bone during swallowing and speech. The bottom illustration demonstrates how unilateral tightness may cause deviation from the midsagital plane.

Action: *With hyoid bone fixed, assists in depressing the mandible to open mouth.*

With mandible fixed, elevates the hyoid bone. Retrudes lower jaw

Inserts: *A. Superior:*
1. *Behind: Mastoid notch deep to attachments of the longissimus capitis, splenius capitis, and SCM*
2. *Anterior: Inferior border of mandible*

B. Inferior: Hyoid bone

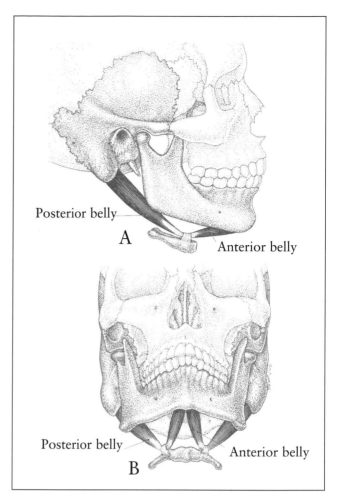

Posterior belly

A

Anterior belly

Posterior belly

B

Anterior belly

Figure 3-121

Figure 3-122. Working with the Mastoid Attachment of the Digastric Muscle

It is not uncommon for the digastric muscle to be tight, especially if your client experiences difficulties in swallowing. Practice palpating the muscle by placing your fingers on the attachments of your own digastric muscle and swallowing. Pulling or pushing the sternocleidomastoid muscle out of the way enables contact with this muscle near its insertion on the mastoid process.

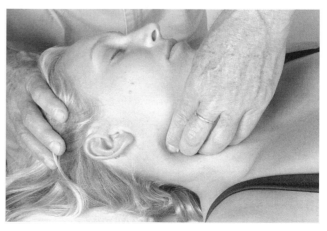

Figure 3-122

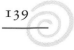

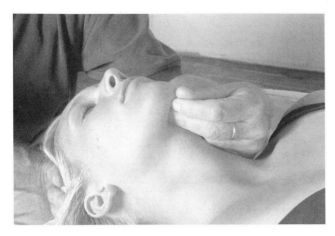

Figure 3-123

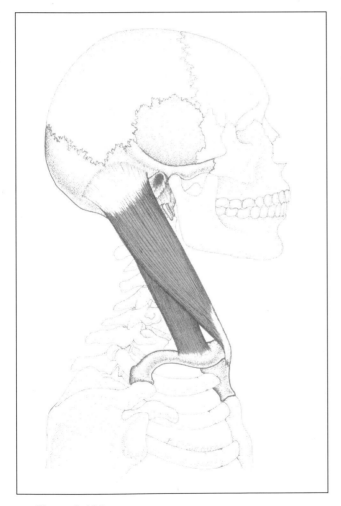

Figure 3-124

Figure 3-123. Working with the Digastric Muscle at the Mandible

Work the attachments at the front of the mandible. Have your client swallow while working, and you will be able to point out tension in the digastric muscle.

Figure 3-124. Anatomy of the Sternocleidomastoid Muscle

This important muscle can be a source of trigger point headaches as well as pain at the mastoid process. When working at the lower attachments, but sure to address both the sternal and clavicular heads.

> *Action: A. Working together, the SCM muscles:*
> > *1. Flex the neck and pull the head forward*
> > *2. Bring chin onto the chest*
> > *3. Assist in inspiration of breath. For thoracic breathers, these muscles may be overdeveloped.*
> > *B. Unilaterally the SCM muscle:*
> > *1. Rotates the face toward the opposite side and tilts it upward*
> > *2. (With the upper trapezius) side-bends the cervical column, drawing the ear to the shoulder*
> *Inserts: A. Above: Mastoid process*
> > *B. Below*
> > *1. Sternal attachment (medial and more superficial)*
> > *2. Clavicular attachment (lateral and deeper)*

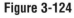

Figure 3-125. Grabbing and Lifting the Sternocleidomastoid Muscle from Deeper Tissue (DVD 5, 1:00:17)

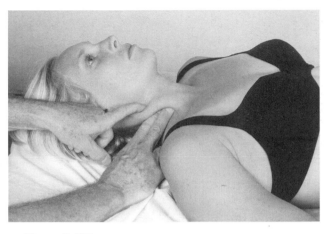

Work the belly of the muscles by using longitudinal strokes and side-to-side mobilization. Lift the belly of the muscle from the deeper muscles and mobilize with small movements. Remember to work the tendinous insertions at the mastoid process.

If the SCM is very tight, for easier access you may need to shorten, rather than stretch it; turning head away from the muscle you are treating will shorten the muscle and make it softer and more easily accessed.

Figure 3-125

Cranial Decompression

Cranial decompression is very useful at the end of a session to provide space between the occiput and the cervicals. It is also useful for returning the nervous system to equilibrium if the client has experienced an autonomic nervous system response during treatment and feels disoriented. If your clients complain of a headache after a session or come in with a headache, this technique often will be helpful to relax the neck enough to reduce or cure symptoms. The biggest error in this technique is to apply too much traction and to tilt the head forward so that the cervical curve is reduced. Most of the pressure should come from the weight of the client's head. Use very little traction and experiment with even compressing the cervicals/occiput a slight bit. Do not attempt to "straighten" the neck by pulling too hard or tilting the head forward. Neck releases are most easily accomplished with the cervicals in a relaxed and neutral position.

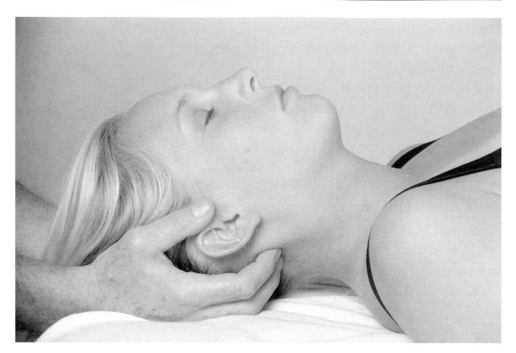

Figure 3-126

Figure 3-126. Cranial Decompression

Force is applied upward at the base of the occiput. Fingers should be slightly curved with most of the force coming from the fleshy tips. The occipital bone should rest in the palm or butt of the hands. Use the sides of the hands and thumbs to gently cradle the head. It will sometimes take several minutes for you to feel the softening associated with decompression.

Chapter Four

Your Role in Looking out for the Health of Your Clients

MANY MASSAGE THERAPISTS, ESPECIALLY THOSE IN PRIVATE PRACTICE, find that their clients respect their views about non-massage health issues and frequently ask advice. This becomes increasingly common as your practice moves towards a more therapeutic or structural nature. Rather than having massage as an occasional luxury, more people are coming to Deep Tissue Massage with the hope of solving problems and, as with diet and exercise, they see it as a component of their routine for a healthy life. They want better athletic performance, more flexibility, emotional release, and the alleviation of pain. They understand the holistic approach to health and may look to you for assistance.

This area can add a rewarding dimension to your work, but also can place you in difficult situations. Over the years, I have encountered some incredible stories of misinformation and downright dangerous advice being offered by well-meaning massage therapists. Some project their own issues onto their clients with unsolicited advice about their clients' personal lives, diet (sometimes even selling health or multilevel marketing products for their own profit), which twelve-step program is needed, or a multitude of other well-intentioned guidance.

Whether or not a massage therapist is qualified to give advice, many clients don't feel close enough to their medical doctors to ask questions about general health, nutrition, psychology, or other disciplines that can greatly impact their lives in a positive way. Thus, the greater your knowledge in tangential health areas, the greater your potential for providing benefit to your clients.

The safest course is to have an extensive list of names for making referrals to experts in a particular area. I have a list of respected osteopaths, chiropractors, orthopedic surgeons, general and homeopathic physicians, podiatrists, acupuncturists, herbologists, nutritional counselors, dermatologists, physical therapists, psychologists, and other health professionals.

I am aware of my own limitations with massage and bodywork. An early teacher of mine quoted the folk wisdom that "if you give a man a hammer, the whole world becomes a nail." I know fellow Rolfers or soft tissue specialists who seem to believe that all pain and physical problems arise from tight muscles or fascia and that softening this tissue is a panacea that only they can provide. The reality is that pain in the body may arise from a multitude of causes, including lack of muscle tone, movement patterns, or serious medical conditions. I frequently refer clients to athletic trainers, Feldenkrais®, Somatics, yoga, Pilates or other movement practitioners. Although I am confident in my manual therapy skills, I also refer to other peers who I feel are more appropriate for the needs of my clients—including other Rolfers or therapists who specialize in particular disorders or disciplines such as trigger point, shiatsu, or athletic massage.

Especially in a fledgling practice, it may be frightening to refer a potential client to someone else, but in the long run, this practice will pay off. Clients will recognize your integrity and concern for their well-being. Also, it is possible that your referral sources will reciprocate your referrals.

Am I advocating that you should never become involved with helping your clients in tangential areas associated with massage? Definitely not! Just be aware of your limitations and remember that it is better to give no information than to give incorrect information. When difficult questions arise, sometimes the best answer is "I don't know."

That caveat having been established, let us explore some of the areas in which you might be interested in providing support for your clients. **(DVD 6, 0:11)**

An Ounce of Prevention

ONE OF THE GREATEST GIFTS YOU CAN GIVE TO CLIENTS is the feeling of empowerment. A large number of the symptoms, even if improved by massage, are the result of improper habits. People feel powerless and accept pain as their lot in life. I recently treated a physician who had never sought treatment for his "bad back" because his father had the same problem and he assumed he "inherited" it. However, that back problem may be a result of improper lifting, poor posture, weakness in muscles that support the back, or countless other causes besides heredity. Massage can certainly help temporarily, but if the poor habits continue, the problems may persist. Holistic or counterculture therapists often, with good cause, criticize the Western medical approach of simply giving pills to alleviate symptoms without looking for causes. However, many of these same practitioners think nothing of trying essentially the same thing with a neverending regime of massage or chiropractic treatments, without attempting to find the source of the problems. Of course, people do have structural issues that receive tremendous benefit from our work, but many of these people could also empower themselves by taking responsibility for pernicious habits and by beginning to trust their own ability to improve their conditions.

One of the first things you can ask is, "What do you think causes the problem?" It is astonishing how few people have had anyone ask this simple question. It is also surprising how many people intuitively know what the cause is but are conditioned into always going elsewhere for help. Chapter Five will deal with therapeutic strategies for specific complaints and will offer strengthening and stretching suggestions for recommending to clients. Expanding your work into this area will earn the respect of your clients and make your practice more interesting, successful, and busy.

The following are very brief listings of possible causes or exacerbating factors in complaints that we often encounter in our massage practices. These causes and solutions may seem simplistic and commonsensical, but you will be amazed at how often clients have not even considered the causes of their problems or have never been given the encouragement to change.

Back Pain

An Old or Improper Mattress—Different people need different amounts of support and comfort when they sleep. Many people assume that the harder the mattress, the better. They sleep on a hard futon that does not accommodate the curves in their bodies. Conversely, sometimes mattresses are just worn out and provide no support.

Weakness in Back and/or Abdominal Muscles—A knowledge of which exercises to suggest is far too complex a subject for this book to cover with more than the most basic suggestions. Even these simple suggestions, which are covered in Chapter Five, have prompted numerous clients over the years to call with thanks for empowering them to cure themselves. I also have had good luck referring clients to physical therapists for a back stabilization program and also have found that Pilates teachers excel in their knowledge of abdominal and low back strengthening protocols.

Chairs and Car Seats that Provide Improper Support, Especially at Work—Clients often report great improvement just from using lumbar support or wedge shaped cushions designed to bring weight onto the ischial tuberosities. Explain the importance of maintaining a proper lumbar curve when seated. Couches are notorious for not supporting the low back; yet people spend hours there while watching television.

Generic Exercises in Classes—Clients sometimes say, "Whenever I do such and such exercise in class, it flares up my back." Yet, they continue to persist because the instructor exhorts everyone to do every exercise. However, different people have different structure, and generic exercise is not for everyone. Some people do well with forward flexion but cannot tolerate extension. Others are just the opposite. This tendency to go on in spite of pain or discomfort is not only common in aerobic or strength classes, but also in yoga and even meditation retreats where there is subtle pressure to sit cross-legged or in the lotus position for long periods of time. One of my clients persists with this practice in spite of the fact that he spends six weeks every year recovering from his one-week meditation retreat.

Poor Postural Habits—I have found clients to be extremely open to changing postural and other habits that contribute to chronic back pain. Most massage classes give instruction about how to roll onto one's side before sitting up to get off of a massage table or to get out of bed in the morning. Although this is important, the majority of us do this only once a day when rousing ourselves to face the day. Most of us get out of chairs countless times a day, and it is surprising how often poor technique in this simple act can create chronic low back problems. I have had countless clients say that learning how to rise from a chair has had the single largest effect on curing chronic back pain. Let's look at the improper (usual) and proper ways of moving from a sitting position to standing.

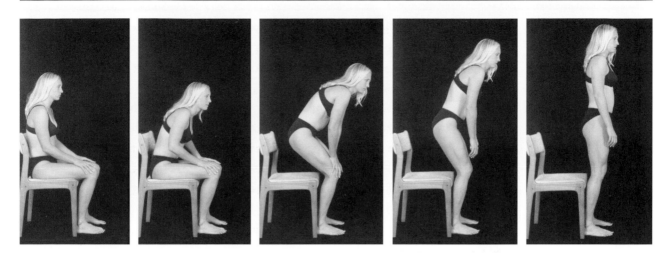

Figure 4-1. Improperly Rising from a Chair

In this example, notice the strain on the lower back. The upper body is bent forward from the waist and the lumbar spine is vulnerable because of forward flexion. Immediately after raising her buttocks from the chair, she must support and then lift half her body weight with her lower back because the legs are not offering support.

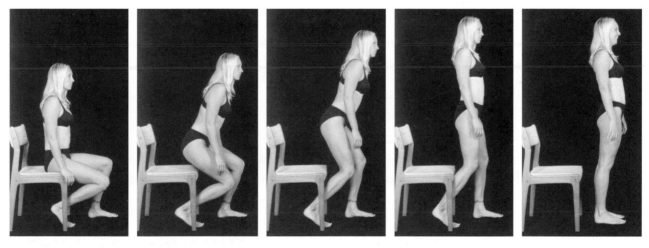

Figure 4-2. Properly Rising from a Chair

Figure 4-2

It is crucial to begin to rise with proper placement of the feet. In this case, the model has moved forward in the seat and has her weight on the sitz bones. Notice that she has placed one foot to the rear and one foot forward for balance, and that the back keeps the proper curve throughout the whole motion. The feet remain under the body during the entire process of rising and the legs provide the energy for rising rather than the lower back.

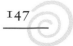

Such simple poor habits as bending forward from the waist to brush teeth or wash dishes, or to rise from bed every morning may cause a chronic back problem. I have had good success in "curing" chronic back problems by giving a few minutes of simple instructions.

One of the most important roles for you as a massage therapist may be to bring your client to a pain-free state by releasing tight muscles, even if it's temporary. If a person is in constant pain, it is often impossible to determine what is causing the pain. But commonly a client may report, "I felt great after the massage until I . . . " Once a person is free from symptoms, he may be able to determine what is causing the pain.

Neck Pain (DVD 7, 13:37)

Prone Sleeping—The strain on the neck due to sleeping on the stomach is a major cause of chronic neck pain. Although it is difficult to break sleeping habits, it is worth the effort.

Choice of Pillow—Many people with neck pain find that using the proper pillow makes a significant difference in resolving the problem. Pillow technology has improved in the last few years giving options of "memory foam" and different density and thickness options. Cervical pillows offer various shapes to provide support to the neck for both side-lying and supine sleepers. I keep several extra pillows on hand to demonstrate to clients and even loan them out for trials. Remember that different people have different needs depending upon their sleeping habits and spinal patterns.

Everyday Habits—From telephone habits and computer use to the tilt of car seats, many people exacerbate neck problems with habitual patterns. Simple changes such as using headphones for extended telephone use, or altering the height of computer monitors can have profound effects.

Weakness and Flexibility Causes—sometimes simple strengthening and flexibility exercises are the answer. Many clients have found that yoga or aerobic or strength training have cured long-standing neck and back problems. However, knowing which exercises to recommend requires study and experience. An exercise that might help ninety per cent of the population can increase symptoms for others. Referring clients to experts is the safest course of action.

Headaches

Even though many people accept them as part of life, chronic headaches are not normal. Causes are complicated and often the result of numerous factors. Muscle tension is frequently a major cause, and precise and focused deep tissue and trigger point massage can be extremely helpful. Other contributing factors can be diet, hormone levels, vision problems, and sometimes more serious medical conditions. It is interesting how many people would rather tolerate frequent headaches rather than examine potential causes such as caffeine or chocolate consumption. Your role might be to temporarily alleviate pain with consistent massage so that they can find what triggers the headache. There is an abundance of literature explaining causes of headaches and offering solutions. This can be an effective method of having your client begin to take responsibility for finding the solution.

More Serious Conditions

LEGALLY, WE ARE NOT ALLOWED TO DIAGNOSE medical conditions or illnesses, and it is not normally our role as massage therapists to advise clients about such things. However, there is one area in which we could possibly save a life. In the past fifteen years, I have alerted three clients about unusual skin growths or moles that, upon medical examination, turned out to be malignant. Skin growths may occur in areas that cannot be seen by your client, or they may assume that a growth is normal. The vast majority of what may appear to be abnormal growths are perfectly safe, so it is extremely important that you do not alarm your client. Simply mentioning the mole or growth and asking if they are aware of it is usually all that is needed. Most people have already had it examined and will appreciate your concern and be impressed with your interest.

Malignant Melanoma

The most deadly skin cancer is malignant melanoma. If suspected, the growth should be examined by a dermatologist immediately. Information and photographs are provided by the American Cancer Society in their pamphlet, *Why You Should Know About Melanoma*. For the good of your clients, please obtain a copy and memorize this information, for early detection of this skin cancer is essential for survival. Some of the most crucial information is reprinted here.

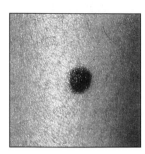

Ordinary mole

◎ What is the difference between a melanoma and an ordinary mole?

An ordinary mole is an evenly colored brown, tan, or flesh colored spot in the skin. It is either flat or raised. Its shape is round or oval and it has sharply defined borders. Moles are generally less than 6 millimeters in diameter (about the size of a pencil eraser). A mole may be present at birth or it may appear later, usually in the first few decades of life. Sometimes several moles appear at about the same time, especially on areas of the skin exposed to the sun. Once a mole has fully developed, it normally remains the same size, shape, and color for many years. Most moles eventually fade away in older persons.

Warning signs: Almost everyone has moles, on the average about 25. The vast majority of moles are perfectly harmless. A change in a mole's appearance is a sign that you should see your physician. However, a melanoma is more complicated than a mole. Here's the simple ABCD rule to help you remember the important signs of melanoma and other skin cancers:

A. Asymmetry. One half of the spot does not match the other half.

B. Border irregularity. Normal moles are round or oval. The borders of a melanoma may be uneven or notched.

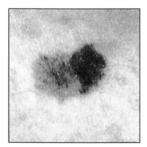

Asymmetry

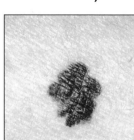

Border irregularity

C. Color. Common moles are usually one color throughout. Melanomas may have several colors or an irregular pattern of colors.

D. Diameter. Common moles are generally les than ¼ inch in diameter (the diameter of a pencil eraser). Melanomas may be ⅛ to ¼ inch, but are often larger.

The most important warning sign is change— a change in size, shape, or color of a spot on your skin.

Other warning signs are:
- A sore that does not heal.
- A new growth.

Most of us have spots on our skin. A benign (non-cancerous) lesion can sometimes look like a skin cancer. Check with your doctor.

Other warning signs of melanoma: Spread of pigment from the border into surrounding skin; redness or a new swelling beyond the border; change in sen-

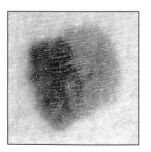

Color

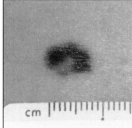

Diameter

sation . . . itchiness, tenderness, or pain. Change in the surface of a mole—scaliness, oozing, bleeding, or the appearance of a lump or nodule.

How is melanoma diagnosed?

If your physician suspects that a change in your skin is a sign of melanoma, a sample of the tissue will be removed. This procedure is called a biopsy, and usually can be done quickly and easily in the physician's office. The tissue sample is then sent to a pathology laboratory for examination under a microscope to confirm the diagnosis.

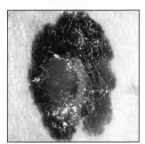

Changes in the surface of a mole

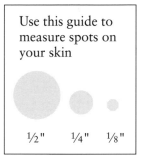

Use this guide to measure spots on your skin

½"   ¼"   ⅛"

Breast Cancer

Next to heart disease, breast cancer kills more women than any other disease. It is good that we are frequently exposed to public service mini-messages on the subject, but it is also common that we hardly notice such sound bytes. It seems that there still is a stigma about talking about breast cancer in one-on-one conversations. Some people feel more at ease talking about the intimacies of their sex lives than about cancer.

I had a wonderful anatomy professor in college, Dr. Marian Diamond, who spent the last day of class lecturing to a class of 250 students about breast cancer. She explained that she thought it was much more important than giving us twenty more anatomy terms that we would forget in a few months. I am sure that she has saved numerous lives over her career by educating her students.

Early detection is essential, and I know several women who discovered malignant breast growths by self-examination. A close relative recently discovered a malignant growth that even a subsequent mammogram failed to detect. Her diligence in performing monthly breast self-exams gave her months of head start on treatment. I am not advocating that you become a crusader in this health issue, but this is a topic in which you could possibly have a profound effect on someone's life. It is a good idea to have an intake form for new clients. Simply asking on this form if your female clients give themselves breast self-exams could be enough to broach the subject or plant a seed for further thought. The American Cancer Society has numerous pamphlets about breast cancer and detailed explanations of how to perform self-examination. Having this information available to give to a client might save a life.

Emotions and Massage

MANY PEOPLE CONSIDER MASSAGE as an important contribution to their mental health. Massage can dissipate emotional stress, and for some people allow contact with repressed emotions. It is not uncommon for clients to be referred to massage therapists by their psychotherapists, who feel that somatic restraints are hindering the therapeutic process.

Any bodywork may act as a catalyst for the release of emotions, but Deep Tissue Massage seems to be associated with more "emotional release" than many other forms of massage. This may be a self-fulfilling prophesy; clients who feel the need for such emotional release may come to a deep tissue practitioner because they feel that they will have permission to experience such a release. Some people feel that receiving a massage just to feel good and receive nurture is self-indulgent, while if they are "working" on emotional issues the work is justified.

The type of work that is effective in releasing emotional holding varies greatly from individual to individual. For most people, being in a safe, non-judgmental environment is the most important component. For some people this may be a gentle, nurturing massage while for others, the intensity of deep work does act as a catalyst. Possibly, the faith required to trust someone to work deeply at a physical level may carry over to an emotional trust. One does not need to subscribe to the theory that emotions are stored in tissue at a cellular level to believe that deep muscular work can be an effective tool to facilitate emotional awareness. Furthermore, if a person has spent his life contracting his chest muscles any time he experiences feelings of sadness, then releasing these muscles may facilitate the release of these emotions.

Often, clients will come for massage and mention the goal of emotional growth or release as a primary reason for being there. Some massage therapists then fall prey to then taking responsibility for this release rather than simply letting whatever comes up happen. If the expected emotional reaction does not occur, the therapist has somehow failed. It is very important to remember that the therapist is only a facilitator and is never responsible for release.

Some therapists have an agenda about emotional issues and judge their effectiveness by whether or not clients experience "emotional release." However, there is great danger in projecting our own values into this area, whether it's judging that release is necessary or that certain emotions are better or worse than others. The emotions of sadness and anger are the most often mentioned, particularly by therapists who are exploring these emotions in themselves. And yet, I have found that a great many clients who have come for emotional release, when allowed to experience what comes up, report that they experience unexpected happiness and a feeling of having the weight of the world lifted from their shoulders. The most important gift you can give is not to judge any emotions that come out in a session and to not try to solve your clients' problems for them.

At the opposite end of the spectrum from clients who anticipate a cathartic release are the persons who are unaware of any link between their body and their emotions. If they start to feel unexpected emotions, they may be frightened and require additional support and explanation to pacify any fear or embarrassment. However, my experience has been that many more people experience a subtle, noncathartic emotional release several days after a deep session rather than during the session. It is sometime a good idea to mention this when you sense that a client may be experiencing an emotional response at an unconscious level.

Stories abound of bodyworkers who are not well-trained in psychological work imposing their emotional belief systems on their clients and playing at being amateur psychologists. Although well intentioned, sometimes such people are simply projecting or acting out their own issues. In most cases, having a referral list of professional psychotherapists is the best idea. This is not to say that the massage therapist should discourage the emotional aspects of the work. As long as we are clear about our role as massage therapists, provide a safe and nurturing environment for our clients, and do not attempt to control the outcome of our work, the emotional aspect can be another interesting and rewarding facet of our profession.

Chapter Five

Therapeutic Strategies for Addressing Common Complaints and Injuries

OST MASSAGE THERAPISTS WHO MAKE THE TRANSITION FROM massage that is primarily relaxation oriented to deep tissue work that addresses painful areas or holding patterns find the work more interesting and fun as well as more rewarding financially. Developing skill in this area is often all that is needed to make the break from "massage mills" where therapists are burning themselves out performing countless carbon copy massages to clients they will never see again. This is not meant to denigrate relaxation-oriented massage or to imply that you must choose one or the other. Many bodywork practices are a blending of these two disciplines. However, if you expand your skills, you will find that you can build a thriving and interesting practice having expertise in multiple areas to compliment your skills in "regular" massage. Your clients will respect the breadth of your knowledge and your referral base will expand.

You should be aware of some of the differences that you will encounter in such a practice. First, you will find that clients with specific complaints will not necessarily expect a full-body massage. Many will prefer slow and focused work on one or two areas. This may seem like common sense, but many students admit that is difficult to break the habits of their first massage class, which taught that it is necessary to work on the entire body in every massage. Performing a full-body massage in a limited amount of time may prevent you from making significant progress with a particular problem because you will be spreading yourself too thin. Try working on a friend or regular client in one area for approximately forty-five minutes or more and see how rewarding it is to address a problem in depth without the time pressure of attempting to cover the whole body.

On the other side of the coin is the tendency to overwork a painful area in an attempt to bring relief. The goal is to offer improvement, not to cure ailments in one session. Don't be cajoled into overworking by compliments about how much better an area feels, but there is still a "little pain or stiffness right here that needs more work." These clients will sometimes call the next day complaining of increased symptoms. It is much better to leave some work uncompleted than to undo the balance you have created by overworking an area. I joke with my friends that they are at risk if they come to me for therapy because I'll try to give them just a little bit extra, resulting in an increase of symptoms.

Troubleshooting Guide

SINCE THE FIRST PUBLICATION OF THIS MANUAL, without a doubt the most growth in the massage industry has been in what I prefer to call "troubleshooting." I choose this term as more inclusive than terms such as "injuries," "medical massage," or "fix-it" work because it covers the treatment of any complaint or desire for improvement in posture or performance that your client may bring to your practice. It also includes the role of the therapist in preventative and maintenance therapy. Just a quick scan of advertisements in any massage publication will demonstrate the abundance of educational materials and workshops promoting techniques that come under this umbrella.

In 2004, *Consumer Reports* conducted a survey of 34,000 members of the public to determine the benefits that different modalities (chiropractic, physical therapy, deep tissue massage, prescribed exercises, prescription medication, acupuncture, acupressure, and diet) provided for various conditions or complaints.* For relieving back pain and neck pain, deep tissue massage was virtually tied with chiropractic for those respondents who felt "much better," and deep tissue work led with those who reported that they felt "somewhat" better. The results were significantly higher than for prescription and over-the-counter drugs and the other modalities, and the statistics are even more impressive when one considers that most chiropractic patients receive multiple sessions per week for extended periods.

---

* "The healing touch," ConsumerReports.org, August 2005.

For fibromyalgia and osteoarthritis, deep tissue massage was the preferred leader for both "significant" and "somewhat better" improvement, although it should be mentioned that physical therapy and exercise were also rated highly. In 2006 the California Chiropractic Association introduced legislation (which failed) that would have limited massage therapists to moving clients within their "voluntary range of motion" and not beyond, which would have made it exceedingly difficult for me to work with a favorite client who has a spinal cord injury. I do find myself asking if there is any correlation between this success in the public perception of the effectiveness of deep tissue massage and the increasing attempts at restricting the scope of practice that conventional medicine and chiropractic are attempting to legislate for our profession. But in any case, massage therapists need to have the knowledge and technical expertise to work appropriately, however defined.

It should also be noted that prescribed exercise consistently rated highly with respondents to the survey. It is crucial for anyone working with injuries or performance to realize that in addition to tightness and adhesions, weakness is often involved in dysfunction and pain. I have had consistent positive feedback from my clients and also from massage therapists who utilize the simple stretching and strengthening exercises in this manual to help educate and empower clients who have imbalances in the body due to weakness or inflexibility. I encourage you to add this dimension to your practice.

Many practitioners feel that adding troubleshooting or problem-solving skills has transformed their practices, both in the enjoyment, and in the financial success of their work. Some therapists would be interested in expanding their practices in this way, but work at a spa or have a clientele who appear to be only interested in relaxation massage, so they don't attempt to bring in these ideas. In reality, many spa clients would love more therapeutic work but are unaware that it is available. It is important to not project possibly false impressions about this subject into your clients, and I know many spa therapists whose major client load comes from people seeking troubleshooting work.

Although it is perfectly legitimate and appropriate for therapists to focus on soothing relaxation work, it is unfortunate if they limit their practice simply because they encounter some difficulty in transitioning to a broader practice. A great deal of the resistance to performing deep and troubleshooting work really doesn't come from a conscious decision but from an unconscious trepidation or confusion about how to make the change. Let's examine some of the factors that may interfere with using deep tissue work to begin working in a problem-solving mode.

Early Training—Beginning massage instruction, by necessity, limits the depth of work and focuses on inculcating proper biomechanics and fundamentals of touch. Early caveats against medicinal approaches to massage are quite wise, but can establish a limiting mind-set that becomes counter-productive as your expertise grows. It may be time to reflect upon how early limits that no longer apply may be restricting your choices, your success in your practice, and your enjoyment of your work.

Confusion About How to Transition—Many therapists are interested in expanding their work to a more therapeutic focus, but imagine that this might bring about too great a change: a quantum leap to suddenly having a string of clients coming in with problems to solve. The reality is that most everyone has something going on in their body that they would happily have improved, even if they primarily want relaxation massage. A considerable number of my clients come for work because their "regular" massage therapist always performs the same massage routine and resists working differently on areas of complaint. The way to transition is to simply gain confidence a little at a time in the more common conditions that respond well to deep work. This can be easily achieved by spending an extra ten or fifteen minutes on problem areas while still performing a traditional massage. It is often an excellent way to have your clients begin booking longer sessions to allow you to concentrate on an area without sacrificing attention to some other area or detracting from the relaxing aspects. There is no need to sacrifice the nurturing work you enjoy just because you expand your expertise.

You may find that certain clients will enjoy the more detailed work so much that they begin scheduling more frequently and coming in for sessions to focus on more detailed "spot work." This is surprisingly easy to accomplish, even in a spa setting where you will develop your own clientele who request you.

Lack of Confidence—This cause may be divided into three subsections:

• *Lack of anatomical knowledge or fear of increasing symptoms:* In classes, as soon as I explain the anatomy of an area we are covering, students relax and grasp the techniques with confidence. Having a good sports medicine book as a reference is an excellent way to brush up on the anatomy and treatment suggestions so as to slowly build confidence.

Of course it is always better to err on the side of caution and not try to "cure" or work with situations when you have limited knowledge. But this knowledge is acquired incrementally. You may begin with relatively easy situations such as a stiff neck, tight IT band, or shoulder immobility. As you gain efficacy and confidence (and possibly after taking a workshop or two), you then may add other areas such as plantar fasciaitis, ribs that are immobile, tennis elbow, pelvic rotational factors, and other increasingly complicated but very interesting and rewarding areas.

• *Belief that there is an accepted and "right" way to work with any specific condition:* Therapists who could do excellent work sometimes are afraid to begin the rewarding incremental acquisition of knowledge because they think that they need to take an expensive workshop to learn the "right" way of working. I often see books and workshops promising specific, step-by-step protocols on how to treat different issues. Sometimes they promise miraculous results and imply that there is only one way to work. However, there are many roads to Rome; that is, many ways to work, depending on the client, the situation, and the skills of the therapist. Simple, cautious, gentle work around a painful area will often relax counterproductive holding patterns and fear, and provide dramatic improvement. Relying upon intuition that has evolved from firm anatomical knowledge and experience is preferable to rote and inflexible protocols.

• *Pressure from Unreasonable Expectations:* Improvement in level of pain or other problems is a complex interplay of multiple factors. Indeed, satisfying the subjective elements of relaxation or enjoyment is typically less demanding than the quantifiable issues of problem solving. Although you may be an important aid or catalyst for improvement, you are not responsible for the results. In classes, I often demonstrate on people with specific complaints. Although it is gratifying to the ego to have great results, I also am very happy to sometimes be less than successful, if for no other reason than to impart the important lesson that not everyone will have extraordinary success with every client. Even the best therapists have a significant number of cases that don't respond with dramatic improvement. When people begin working on troubleshooting, the most common error is to expect too much of oneself and to assume that someone else would probably "know what to do" and be successful. An excellent segue into such work is, "Let's see if I can provide some help here." Less than 100 percent success is not a sign of failure.

Another way to remove pressure from yourself is to let discretion be the better part of valor and feel free to say "I don't know" if you do not have a clear idea of how to deal with an issue. We are not expected to know everything about every condition, and referral to another practitioner is often wise and appreciated by your clients.

Dealing with Red Tape and Insurance—This can indeed be a problem, and some therapists choose to not get involved in legal or insurance cases. But many therapists really have no idea how to work in this domain and that it is easier than suspected. A section later in this chapter will provide some details and understanding of this subject.

Treating the Person and Not Just the Injury

Injuries and pain do not exist in a vacuum; they are the results of often complex causes and cannot be separated from the infinite complexity that is a human being. When dealing with troubleshooting work, your first contact with the person will set the stage for how you plan your work, an ongoing relationship, and the possible outcomes of treatment. Even if you specialize in relaxation massage, it is a good idea to schedule at least fifteen minutes of extra time for first-time clients to establish a relationship. You will be surprised what will come out of the mouths of complete strangers if you simply sit down with them for a few minutes and ask what they are looking for in a massage. This is often a way to clarify therapeutic goals and to educate the client on the advantages of detailed work rather than superficial work spread out over the entire body. It also gives the client a chance to begin to trust and establish a bond with you. On pages 214–215 is a sample intake form. A brief intake will present you in a more professional light, and some therapists mail a questionnaire to clients before the first session, which also may prevent the dreaded first session cancellation syndrome.

Some productive questions and discussion prompts would be:

What other treatments have you tried? What have been most helpful and what have not?

Are you taking any medications for this? This question also opens the door for clients to offer any other medications they may be taking for other issues that might have importance. If over-the-counter pain medication helps, it can give you an idea about their threshold of pain. Often clients are unaware of the differences between medications that decrease inflammation at the site of pain such as non-steroidal anti-inflammatory drugs (NSAIDS) and those that affect the body's sensation of pain at the central nervous system such as acetaminophen or stronger narcotics. Of course we must show caution in discussing medication choices with clients and should not make recommendations, but educating them on the cost/benefit decisions involved in such choices will often be welcomed.

Frequently inflammations are self-perpetuating, and treating with NSAIDS will help break this cycle rather than just dull the perception of pain in the brain while allowing the inflammation to continue. With good reason, many clients are reluctant to take pain medication, but it is important to consider that the body's compensatory reactions to pain may complicate and prolong the recovery to acute injuries.

Regardless of the type of medication, if your client is taking any pain medication, but especially stronger varieties with narcotic effects, you will have to adjust the intensity of your work to compensate for this. If your client reports receiving a steroid (cortisone) injection, work at the site of the injection is contra-indicated for at least two weeks. You may have to consider whether they have a strong attachment to the pain medication, which may cause them to focus on their pain in order to justify the medication—this would fall under the "secondary gain" category.

What do you think caused the trouble? Whether athletic pursuits, work, or posture, the cause of the problem is almost always worthy of discussion. Sometimes the most simple suggestions such as using a telephone headset, a lumbar support pillow, altering an athletic training regimen, learning how to rise from a chair, carrying a different type of purse can have a dramatic effect and may not have been considered by the client. It is often unrealistic to expect even the best work to solve problems caused by improper use of their bodies.

Is the condition chronic or acute? Most therapists are apprised of this distinction. Acute problems must be treated more gingerly until the body's initial inflammatory reactions stabilize. In this stage, work that initially gives relief while being performed may actually re-stimulate the inflammatory process and increase symptoms after the session. Most often, ice is beneficial, both after the session and frequently throughout the day. Chronic conditions that are stable may respond better to heat and more aggressive treatment, in large part because the client will have experience in knowing what is an appropriate amount of work.

Another distinction that is useful is that a condition can be "chronic-acute." In this case, what appears to be a chronic condition is actually a recurrent acute inflammation that is activated each time the client performs a certain daily activity. It can be a "bad" back that is activated each time someone gets out of bed or a chair improperly, lifts with improper posture, or trains improperly for an athletic event. Spending time to figure out the activity that causes the pain is a worthwhile endeavor to begin to correct the problem. The cause of pain is often difficult to determine, especially if pain is present at all times. Even temporary relief offered by your treatment may enable your client to determine the cause of pain as it suddenly is activated after a pain-free period. In these cases, frequent application of ice is often helpful, even though most advice suggests only ice for acute inflammation.

Does the problem worsen or get better throughout the day or with exercise? Tendonitis often improves as an area warms up throughout the day. Problems that are associated with weakness or improper postural or work habits may tend to worsen as the day progresses and fatigue sets in. Of course tendonitis may also be associated with weakness, but strengthening and stretching may be suggested, depending upon how the symptoms manifest themselves.

Does the problem improve or worsen with active and passive motion testing? If a client mentions pain with a specific movement such as raising an arm through a certain range of motion, it is a good idea for you to try passively moving the arm through the same range of motion to see if it changes the symptoms. If the pain disappears with passive movement, then the contraction of muscles creating the movement is involved, and weakness may be a factor. If the pain remains in passive movement, then one has to consider the possible structural factors in the joint.

How does it benefit you to suffer from this condition? Of course you can't ask the client this question, but reading between the lines may be helpful. If the client has either a conscious or unconscious benefit from their complaint, it may impede their improvement. This is definitely not implying that they are malingering or being dishonest. But if a Workers' Compensation claim or auto accident is involved or countless other complicating factors, including the emotional makeup of the client and his relationship with his friends or family, then the effects of your treatment will be influenced. This is not to say that you should shun working with such cases or try to delve into deep psychological matters, but it is important to not expect too much of yourself in the improvement of complicated cases.

How might your emotional state influence your symptoms? Again, it is important not to attempt to provide psychological counseling for your clients. With pain in particular, feelings of sadness, depression, anger, and fear can greatly influence the perceptions of your client about the progress they are making. Fear is a particularly important emotion as people assign meaning to their symptoms—"I can no longer ..." "I may lose my ..." "What if ..." These feelings can hypersensitize the person to their problems. I am extremely careful to err towards caution in bringing up such issues, but also feel that a nurturing and genuinely caring openness to listening can often be a tremendous gift, and one that is often missing in conventional allopathic treatment.

Planning Your Session

The tone and scope of your session can be well-defined without being scripted. Different people will have different goals—some realistic and some not. After taking the history, one of the easiest ways to achieve clarity and continuity is simply to ask what they would like from you and what they would hope for in the work, and then to define the limits that you feel are appropriate. It is important to have realistic goals—not to provide false optimism—but remember that hope is often instrumental in recovery.

Lack of success in troubleshooting is often a result of trying to accomplish too much and overworking an area. Establish your goals and work plan early and don't get carried away by your client's comments about how good the work is feeling and requests for "just a little more work there." You goal should be to improve the situation, not cure it. It is always best to err towards the side of caution. A slow steady improvement is almost always the best course, rather than two steps forward and one step back.

However, if your client reports increased symptoms, there is no need to run for the hills. This happens to everyone occasionally, but rarely means that you have damaged the area. Sometimes mentioning that you have released held tension or adhesions and that this may increase symptoms temporarily is all that is needed to allay any fear that your client may have.

If your client expresses a complaint about their body or pain in a particular area, try to determine global issues in their body that may be influencing the situation. This holistic approach is very well explained in Tom Myers' *Anatomy Trains* and in his excellent workshops. If clients experience pain in the rhomboids, try to determine if that is in response to a primary tightness elsewhere, such as the chest, that may causing the reaction as a compensation.

Clients will often be protective of painful areas, and it is sometimes counterproductive to dive in where they are most sensitive and fearful. Rather than trying to massage away localized pain, it is often a good idea to begin work in a satellite area that is not too sensitive or protected and slowly expand that area into the painful area.

Your clients will always want the quickest improvement possible and will often want a timetable of expected benefits. Although it is good to have some motivation for progress, this desire to gauge their progress by some arbitrary timetable is counterproductive. Clients may push themselves too hard or wonder what is wrong if their expectations are not met. I never hazard a guess about when an injury will be "back to normal." It is rewarding to see the look of relaxation on a client's face as they let go of their feelings of counterproductive anxiety and pressure to "perform" by comparing their recovery with that of others or with some ideal.

Feel free to discuss a treatment plan with your clients. It is not realistic to see someone an hour every week or two and expect miraculous improvement—especially when they may be continuing to exacerbate their problem between visits. Sometimes scheduling more frequent and shorter sessions will enable a steady improvement and remove the pressure of trying to accomplish too much at one time and overworking an area.

Ask your client if they are interested in working on the problem on their own by strengthening, stretching, and other productive measures. Some will simply prefer to be treated with your deep tissue expertise, but others will be surprised and thankful for any suggestions you might have. Particularly for stubborn problems like plantar fasciaitis, frozen shoulders, and specific tendonitis, I often get grateful calls from clients who are excited with their improvement between visits as they empower themselves by working on the issues themselves. Remember that we cannot diagnose medical conditions, but your growing expertise in working with problems will improve your professionalism and create word-of-mouth business.

Do you have a network of referrals for problems that you feel could be helped by someone else with a different expertise? This referral should not be based upon a quid pro quo reciprocity, although such beneficial relationships will often naturally occur.

The Intangibles—Your Healing Manner

Before continuing with the specifics of treating the common conditions that one encounters in a massage practice, a few words are in order about the subjective aspects of your relationship with your clients. The most common com-

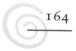

plaint I hear about the conventional Western medical treatment concerns the dehumanizing atmosphere. Patients are often made to feel like they are just a set of symptoms and are almost an imposition on the medical provider as they are rushed from one specialist to another and often just given some pills to take. But this conception is by no means universal and before continuing, I do feel it important to state that I have experienced a great deal of excellent and sincerely caring treatment from the medical community.

The fact remains that a relationship of trust and caring is a huge factor in the outcome of treatment. As massage becomes more scientifically based and accepted by the medical community, I feel that it is critical that we not sacrifice the very qualities that have helped our effectiveness by imitating the negative points of the medical system in the effort to appear more professional. From years of teaching, I am convinced that massage therapists are among the most generous and compassionate group of people in existence. We are exceptionally lucky that we can feel and express that in such a rewarding profession.

Your relationship with your client can be the intangible variable that will bring success to your treatment. The best techniques may not prove effective if performed in a cold, impersonal manner. Probably the most important gift you can give your clients is to allow them to feel like a person rather than a set of symptoms or an allotted time segment in your busy day. To do this, I've learned that listening is one of the most effective tools—and not just listening to the specifics of their complaints. A few simple conversational questions about work, family, interests may open a healing connection that is missing in a more sterile environment.

Over the years I can honestly say that, although I have sometimes been sorely tested, I sincerely like and genuinely care for all my clients. In varying degrees, I have a relationship with each as a person rather than just as a paying customer. If you can convey that you sincerely care for your client, offer a positive and supportive atmosphere where they can be themselves and feel safe to experience and say what they feel, you may provide the ideal environment for healing to take place.

Red Tape

I recently heard another massage therapist scoff at a colleague by declaring that, "… she doesn't even know how to write SOAP notes." (We will cover this subject shortly so you won't have to worry about being ostracized by peers who are more apprised of medical jargon.) Whether it is SOAP notes, intake forms, or dealing with insurance companies, many therapists are put off by the hoops that must be jumped through if one is dealing with medical, legal, governmental (Workers' Compensation), or personal insurance realms and requirements.

There are, of course, certain vocabulary and established communication practices, but these are easily learned and should not discourage you if you are interested in working with these systems. This can be a long and complicated subject and there are a fair number of books and software options to help you out if you look for advertisements in massage magazines or on the Internet. It is not the domain of this book to provide all the details for working with third-party payments, but I will cover the subject briefly in the hope that the subject will become less intimidating. Samples of intake forms, liens, SOAP notes, and a billing template are included at the end of this chapter as examples that you can adapt to your own preferences or duplicate for your use.

Both for your information and for a professional impression, an intake form is an excellent idea, even if it is only for your own use. Some forms are quite formal and ask detailed questions about specific medications, emotional and psychological state, use of recreational drugs, and other personal issues. Although this may be a good idea, my personal preference is to err towards not being too invasive in personal matters. Our scope of practice is much more limited than that of a medical doctor, and such information may be viewed by your client as too personal or even pretentious.

Whatever intake form you utilize, you should allow plenty of time on the first visit for the client to fill out the form and to allow for discussion. You may want to mail the form to the client before the first visit; this can save time, allowing the client to be thorough, and establish a relationship of sorts before the first visit. If you state your cancellation policy on the form, you will appear professional and insure that the client will respect your boundaries. Having the anatomical cartoons in the sample intake form is an excellent way for the client to be able to clearly indicate what areas are bothersome, and save you the embarrassment in follow-up sessions of having to ask which side of the body is experiencing the symptoms.

A medical lien is sometimes used in personal injury or occasional Workers' Compensation cases as a legal guarantee that you will receive a share of any awards after the case settles. The form provided on page 216 is universally acceptable, although it might be a wise idea to make a quick call to your client's attorney to verify that everything is in proper legal order.

The aforementioned SOAP notes are the accepted way of charting work on a client each session in a medical setting. Often, insurance companies or attorneys will ask for your notes. The acronym stands for the following:

S = Subjective—These include the complaints and symptoms as described by the client. This may include personal feelings about past or present causes or the impact upon their lives and what increases or decreases symptoms. Having the client rate their pain on a scale of one to ten is helpful to chart progress of treatment. The amount of detail can vary, but I am careful to not include extraneous information that may be misused by insurance companies or attorneys trying to place cause or blame on other parties in an attempt to escape their responsibility.

O = Objective—These are the observations of the practitioner and include specific visual or tactile observations such as location of pain, spasm, adhesions, or trigger points upon palpation; weakness; range of motion restrictions or pain; postural patterns; etc. Some of your observations might be appropriate for the next category (Assessment), but comparisons to previous descriptions to show progress are fine in the Objective section.

A = Assessment—These comments may be a combination of the two previous sections but are confined to the immediate reactions to the treatment during or after the therapy. This may include objective measurement of range of motion or perception of pain. Because insurance companies often refuse to pay for palliative treatment (other than medication) and require progress in resolving an issue, quantifiable improvement is often stated in this section.

P = Plan—This section addresses suggestions for future treatment such as frequency, different modalities, and home strengthening and stretching suggestions. It is often a good idea to remind yourself of suggestions for future work that may not have been addressed in the current session.

Some more detail here may help you. SOAP notes may be as short as a few brief sentences or quite detailed. For your own use, it is suggested that you have fairly detailed notes to help your memory for returning clients. Although I used the SOAP protocol when working at a physical therapy office, I have not used this form in my private practice and have submitted my less formal notes to legal and insurance companies for years without any problems. SOAP

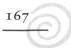

notes that are submitted for legal purposes need not be typed; your original handwritten notes are perfectly acceptable and do not need to be re-copied. See the example below.

S: Jennifer returns 5 days after last treatment on 1/10/07. Reports a slow improvement in L. shoulder pain and notices that driving the car is much easier with reduced pain in the A/C joint. She rates pain level as vacillating between a five and a seven during the day. 3 days after last treatment, while carrying groceries she had a sudden "twinge" in the posterior shoulder and increased symptoms in the posterior capsule for about 36 hours, but felt much better yesterday and continues to improve. Her attitude remains optimistic. She does her exercises with yellow Theraband 2x daily and thinks the external rotation and supraspinatus strengthening and the internal rotation stretches are very helpful.

O: Her range of motion steadily improving in both internal and external rotation with arm abducted to 90 degrees. Is now 15 degrees short of full external rotation in abduction and 23 degrees short in internal rotation. Supraspinatus and infraspinatus are still fibrous and sensitive to palpation and she has a trigger point in R. upper trap that refers to her R. temple – but no real headaches now. Still quite weak in external rotation compared to her L. arm, possibly due to inhibition and protection due to pain.

A: Began with 10 minutes of heat and am able to work more intensely with myofascial release and joint mobilization than last week. PNF stretches for internal and external rotation continue to be effective and she releases more quickly now. Still feels fatigue with yellow Theraband with 3 sets of 10 reps and not ready for a heavier band until pain levels decrease. Reports a little soreness in the areas we worked, but this is common. Fifteen minutes of ice after treatment.

P: Since Jennifer has a tendency to lose mobility after 4 or 5 days, treatment should continue at 2x weekly for at least a couple more weeks as she continues to stretch with more ease in her home program. As inflammation decreases, will increase strengthening exercises and begin pulley exercises next week and possibly add exercises to strengthen in abduction above her shoulders. Remains protective and restrained in her movement, and we discussed that as long as she is careful, she needs to work through the pain a little to improve mobility

Billing

This can be a complicated and extensive issue. There are excellent books explaining the intricacies and software programs that will enable you to have up-to-date information about the codes that are accepted with insurance and legal cases. Since regulations vary from state to state and are constantly changing, this section will deal with the general issues to give the reader a broad understanding. A typical billing template is provided at the end of this chapter.

The important thing to understand is that most insurance companies require CPT (Current Procedural Terminology) codes that represent the particular treatment you are performing—for example: 97124 stands for massage, while 97140 refers to manual therapy techniques. Depending upon how long you work and what combination of procedures you utilize, the process of billing can become a daunting process. Different codes pay different amounts for each 15-minute segment, and additional 15-minute segments may be paid for at a lesser rate. I rarely have trouble when I simply state the code and the total time spent and my normal charges for that time period. Different states have different amounts that they pay for the amount and type of therapy performed. Although you may be able to find out that upper limit of payment, it is easier to simply bill your rate and accept any reductions that the companies may impose.

When I first began bodywork, everyone was excited about the future possibility of insurance coverage of massage. Unfortunately, the amount of work and frustration of dealing with insurance issues (both personal and Workers' Compensation), and to a lesser extent, personal injury claims from auto and other injuries, has left many therapists throwing in the towel in frustration. However, many therapists who have mastered dealing with the system have full practices focusing on this area. If you are serious about performing "third party" recovery work, it may be worth your time to purchase billing software or to take advantage of a professional billing service.

If an occasional insurance case is all you deal with, however, don't be intimidated by the process. It can provide substantial income and provide an interesting array of troubleshooting possibilities as well as providing much-needed help to clients who aren't responding to medication or other treatments. This may sound cynical, but I sometimes have pondered the possibility that insurance companies may actually not want to pay benefits and attempt to frustrate providers by frequently losing bills or underpaying. Just be sure to dot your "i's" and cross your "t's" or your bill will likely be sent back to you to be re-submitted. It is imperative that you have a diagnosis code for the injury and a proper CPT code for treatment. Also, most insurance companies require a tax ID number or your Social Security number on the statement.

The above information about the red tape involved in working with insurance claims may seem complicated at first and will necessitate some trial-and-error learning. You may find that most of your clients are perfectly happy to pay out of pocket for your expert care. The important thing is that you not limit yourself in providing the best care possible just because of discomfort in dealing with such matters. Your skill in working with troubleshooting issues will prove essential to having a thriving and interesting practice regardless of how you deal with insurance.

Applications

Although there will be some overlap, the suggestions for Deep Tissue Massage in this chapter are more specific than the general directions of earlier chapters. Often, you will use the same strokes you would use in a full-body massage, but will work more meticulously to find precise areas of spasm, fibrosis, or emotional holding to patiently open an area.

The same symptoms in different people may have different causes that will benefit from different treatments. Flexibility may be the primary source of some people's problems, while weakness may be a problem for others. These general protocols are simple and safe, but if you find yourself drawn to this type of treatment, you may want to purchase some sports medicine texts for more detailed descriptions of both injuries and treatment protocols.

The following protocols also offer flexibility and strengthening suggestions, which may prove to be the missing link in healing. As mentioned earlier, many injuries are a result of weakness or inflexibility, and it is unrealistic to expect a single massage to correct this imbalance by itself. A large number of clients will be enthusiastic to perform simple exercises to improve their conditions between massage treatments.

When offering suggestions for a home program for your clients, it is important that you ascertain their willingness to take responsibility for their recovery. It is perfectly natural that some clients may just wish to receive your deep tissue skills without committing to exercises. If they express an interest, it is a good idea to ask how much time and effort they are willing to commit and to not overwhelm them with too many suggestions.

If there is significant inflammation, begin with the flexibility exercises and work up to strengthening suggestions as the inflammation subsides. Add exercises incrementally so you can determine their effect. If you give five exercises at one time, four of them may be perfect, but the fifth might increase symptoms. It is then impossible to determine what caused the flare up. Also, begin with the simplest and move to more difficult and complex exercises. Remember that if a stretch or strengthening exercise seems to increase symptoms, it may actually indicate a weakness or inflexibility. The exercises may be beneficial but simply need to be performed with less weight or fewer repetitions.

The growing popularity of disciplines such as Pilates, Feldenkrais® and other movement training, yoga, and memberships to health spas, is an indication of the willingness of our clients to take responsibility for their healing. If you take the time to learn some simple suggestions for your clients' well-being, your practice can become even more rewarding and profound.

◎ Most injuries to the extremities will be to only one side of the body; however, it is recommended to perform strengthening and stretching exercises to both sides. Some astute students have questioned if performing, for example, exercises to both legs when only one knee is injured might overstrengthen the healthy knee and create an imbalance. Actually, the uninjured knee will need to be a bit stronger in order to compensate for the weakness in the other side. Studies also demonstrate that the weak leg will increase strength more quickly than the normal leg because the amount of weight that is used will be more taxing for the weaker muscles, so they will improve at a faster rate. You may want to recommend that more sets be performed on the injured side, however. The other benefit of performing bilateral strengthening is that you will have a comparison to tell you when both sides are equal in strength.

The Ankle (DVD 6, 17:19)

THE ANKLE IS ONE OF THE MOST FREQUENTLY INJURED AREAS that we see as massage therapists. Sprains are the most common injury, and massage is very useful in speeding the early healing process by increasing circulation and reducing swelling. Clients will sometimes call immediately after spraining an ankle and ask for massage. In most cases, the best treatment is to delay soft tissue work until after the initial acute inflammation has subsided. Depending upon the extent of injury, this may be as early as one day or over a week. Immediately after injury, the safest advice you can give your client is to elevate the ankle, use compression to reduce swelling, and to ice frequently.

◎ Caution: Even an apparent slight sprain may be masking a fracture, so the safest course both for healing and for liability reasons is to suggest an x-ray. Most ankle sprains are not serious, but one rare situation should be mentioned: The most commonly injured ligament injury in ankle sprains is the anterior talofibular ligament, which connects the lateral malleolus to the talus bone. Although rare, in severe sprains, this ligament may remain intact, but be pulled from its attachment at the fibula or talus. Often, the client will have heard a loud "pop" at the injury site. Although the goal of most therapy for sprained ankles is to restore normal movement to the ankle, in this case it is very important to immobilize the ankle so that the ligament can reattach. If you have any doubts, require an x-ray before moving the ankle.

When you feel it is safe to work on a sprained ankle, if there is still considerable swelling or discoloration, the most benefit will be derived from effleurage to increase circulation and reduce swelling. Work should not be painful to your client. Next, proceed to deeper work and slow gentle movement to increase mobility and overcome the *splinting* response that immobilizes the ankle. The most benefit from Deep Tissue Massage will be accomplished from one to several weeks after the injury, depending on the severity. If your client has been limping for an extended time period, you will need to perform detailed deep tissue work at areas that are impeding normal motion. Work to retune the inversion/eversion balance and to have the plantar/dorsi flexion be smooth and in a straight line in relation to the tibia.

Soft Tissue Strategies

Figures 5-1a and b. Releasing the Anterior Leg and Calf Muscles

Begin by returning normal function above the ankle; both the anterior and posterior leg will be stiff. The tibialis anterior in the front and the gastrocnemius and soleus in the calf may have become inflexible because the ankle was unable to flex. In both prone (having the feet hanging over end of or the side of the table) and supine position, first passively extend the foot, feeling for

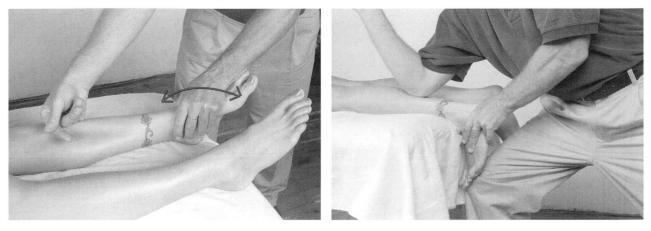

Figure 5-1a

Figure 5-1b

areas where the tissue is hard or bunched and concentrating work in these areas. After passively moving the foot and ankle, ask the client to actively flex and extend the foot; this helps retrain proprioceptive responses so that limping habits are extinguished.

Figures 5-2 a and b. Softening the Achilles Tendon (DVD 6, 30:06)

The Achilles tendon will often be affected in an ankle sprain. It may have been twisted in the original accident, or may become stiff because of ankle immobility during recovery. Work on either side of the Achilles tendon with your fingers or knuckles while "crimping" the Achilles sheath to restore flexibility.

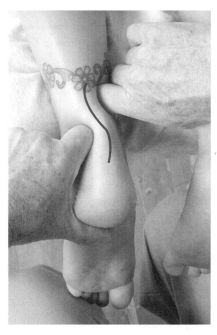

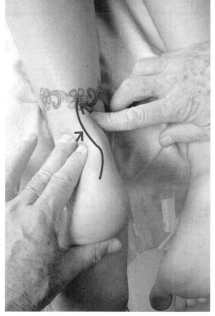

Figure 5-2a

Figure 5-2b

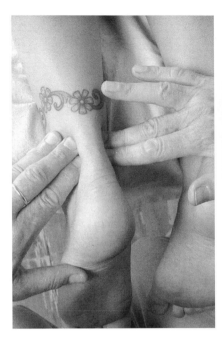

Figure 5-3

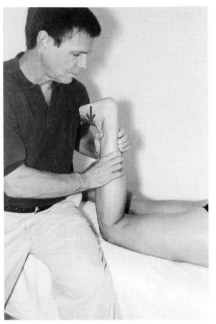

Figure 5-4

Figure 5-3. Lifting the Achilles Tendon from Deeper Tissue

This demonstrates a technique to contact the anterior aspect of the tendon and lift it up away from the tibia.

Figure 5-4. Stretching the Posterior Compartment in Prone Position

By placing your client's forefoot in your axilla area, it is possible to work with both hands and to stretch the calf by applying pressure to the ball of the foot with your own weight.

Working in Gravity (DVD 6, 33:38)

Joints behave very differently when they are treated in a weight-bearing position, which approximates the more natural forces to which they are exposed. You will find that it is very effective to occasionally have your client stand to perform deep tissue work on an area. You will be able to quickly determine areas of restriction, and your clients will immediately notice the effectiveness of your work.

Figure 5-5. Standing Ankle Retinaculum Work

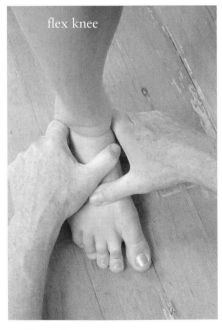

flex knee

Figure 5-5

The foot will often be limited in its ability to flex at the front of the ankle where it articulates with the tibia. To check for limitations to mobility, have your client stand and flex her knee forward while keeping the heel down in the same manner used to stretch the soleus muscle, which will be shown in Figure 5-10. This also will inform her of remaining restrictions and the benefits of your work as she notices the improved flexibility. Anchor the retinaculum or any areas that seem to be restricting movement and ask the client to bend the knee forward to end range while keeping her heel down.

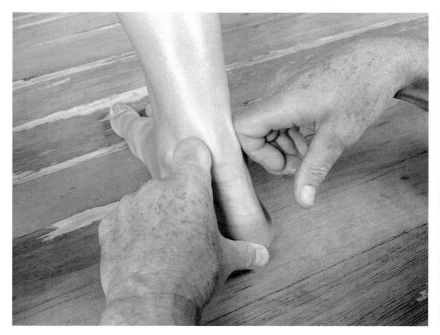

Figure 5-6a

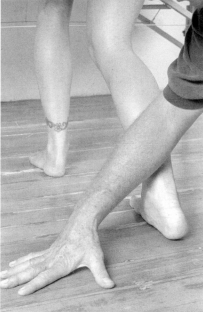

Figure 5-6b

Figures 5-6 a and b. Standing Achilles Tendon and Calf Work

Work the Achilles tendon with fingers or knuckles and the gastro-cnemius and soleus with the forearm while asking for flexion and extension of ankle.

Strengthening Strategies

Figure 5-7. Strengthening Ankle Eversion (DVD 6, 17:25)

Although inversion is also helpful, strengthening the muscles of eversion should be the most important goal because these are the muscles that are needed to stabilize the ankle and prevent reinjury. Notice that the knee is flexed at a right angle and stabilized by the client so that all the movement occurs at the ankle rather than at the hip or knee. Use elastic tubing that can be purchased at any medical supply store in different resistance strengths. Begin with the ankle inverted and slowly evert. Begin with five repetitions, and increase to three sets of ten repetitions.

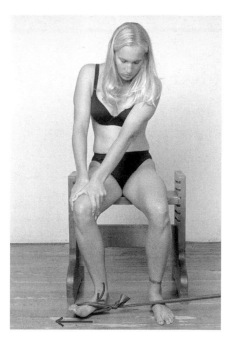

Figure 5-7

 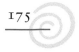

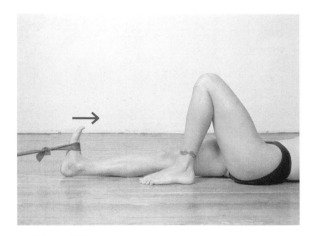

Figure 5-8

Figure 5-8. Strengthening Ankle Dorsiflexion

To strengthen the anterior compartment, the client should anchor the foot in plantar flexion and dorsiflex against resistance, working up to three sets of ten.

For plantar flexion you may instruct your client to hold the tubing above the ankle and extend the foot away from resistance. However, usually simple toe raises will work fine. Begin with both legs and progress to one-legged toe raises. The goal of rehabilitation should be equal strength when performing toe raises unilaterally.

Stretching Strategies

Figure 5-9. Gastrocnemius Stretch

The wall push-up primarily stretches the gastrocnemius of the posterior leg. Instruct clients to have feet comfortably balanced with the heel of the posterior leg anchored to the floor, and then to slowly bend forward with the knee straight until a stretch is felt in the calf.

It is also effective to stand with the forefoot on a step and let the heel slowly drop an inch or two below the foot, allowing the other leg to support some of the weight so that the calf is not overstretched. Although rare, there is a danger that stretching that far could strain or even rupture the Achilles tendon.

Figure 5-10. Soleus Stretch

Having the back knee bent will isolate the soleus muscle and focus the stretch at the soleus muscle and the Achilles tendon. Rather than bringing the whole body forward as in the previous example, have clients just slowly bend the knee forward towards the wall while keeping the heel on the floor.

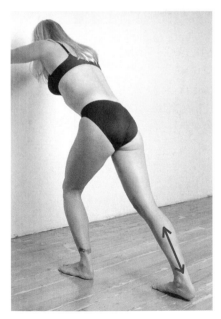

Figure 5-9

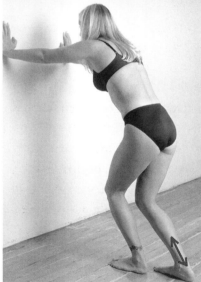

Figure 5-10

Figure 5-11. Alternative Soleus Stretch

Placing the ball of the foot on a two-by-four or similar prop will focus even more stretch on the Achilles tendon and soleus muscle. Instruct clients to slowly bend the knee forward while the foot is on the prop.

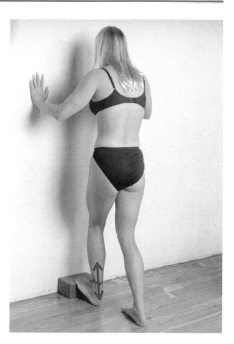

Figure 5-11

Plantar Fasciaitis (DVD 6, 24:12 and 30:06)

PLANTAR FASCIAITIS SEEMS TO BE GROWING in popularity as a diagnosis, especially since several sports celebrities have suffered from this ailment. However, it is by no means limited to athletes; most clients that I see with this problem are over forty-five and many are not athletic. This condition is particularly disruptive to the lives of older clients who must curtail physical and rewarding social activities because of the pain on the plantar surface of the feet, particularly at the front of the heel. Massage has proven to be extremely effective in treating this ailment.

It should be mentioned that some of the suggestions for treatment that follow differ from the conventional conservative medical advice. The common medical advice is for rest and discontinuation of any activity that causes symptoms. Patients are instructed always to wear shoes so that the foot is cushioned and remains in a relatively neutral position. Sometimes cortisone injections or nonsteroidal medication will be prescribed. For relatively new cases, this often is successful, but the symptoms may return when normal activity is resumed. The pain is caused by tight and inflexible plantar fascia and, also by tight calf muscles. Medication and rest may improve symptoms, but if the causes are not addressed, the likelihood of reoccurrence is increased.

Students report an extremely high success rate in treating plantar fasciaitis, especially when the clients perform the simple home regimens of plantar fascia softening and stretching regularly. As important as deep tissue work to the plantar fascia is, it is unrealistic to expect a session every week or two to resolve the tightness causing the pain. Clients who are proactive and willing to see you for treatment regularly and frequently and also perform home exercises are the most successful in curing the problem.

Soft Tissue Strategies

Use the same techniques shown earlier for treating the plantar surface of the foot (Figures 3-7, 3-8, 3-9), but work much more slowly and carefully. Remember that that areas of most acute pain at the front of the calcaneus are reacting to tightness both in the forefoot and the calf. Spend more time in these areas rather than directly at the point of pain.

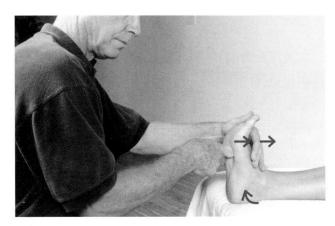

Figure 5-12

Figure 5-12. Treating Plantar Fasciaitis

It is crucial to stretch the tissue rather than using too much lubricant and just rolling over tight areas. Use your other hand to flex the ankle and the toes to provide more stretch. Be careful to not work too aggressively; inflammation may not show up until the next day. Increase intensity after determining how the client tolerates the work. Instruct clients to ice the area after they leave or, better yet, apply ice for ten minutes while you work elsewhere.

Stretching Strategies

Since the pain is primarily in the heel, people often bear weight on their forefeet in an attempt to keep weight off the heel. This further tightens and shortens the calf muscles and exacerbates the problem. The calf stretches shown in Figures 5-9, 5-10, and 5-11 are very important and should be performed several times a day. Ask clients not to stretch first thing in the morning but to allow the area to warm up first with normal activity. Although clients are often instructed always to wear soft shoes around the house, I find that they often become dependent upon the shoes and that the slightest deviation from this practice becomes painful. Of course it is important to not further inflame the area, but enabling the foot to gradually encounter the different positions of walking without shoes can hasten a return to normal activities.

Softening the plantar fascia is most important. Have your client roll their foot on a golf ball or Footsie Roller several times a day to keep the fascia soft and pliable. Freezing an empty soda bottle to roll the foot on is also helpful. Ice the area after any therapeutic activities that might inflame the area, and ice anytime it is convenient—especially before bed.

For more severe cases, podiatrists can be very helpful by designing orthotics or teaching the patient to tape the foot. Before trying this alternative, your client may want to try using "heel cups" which are available at most sporting goods stores.

Plantar fasciaitis is a notoriously slow healer. Work with your client to keep a positive attitude and not give up. Some therapists find it difficult to suggest more frequent treatment, but it is important to consistently soften the tissue and work for steady improvement rather than waiting until symptoms increase before seeking treatment. If your client is hesitant to commit to full-length massage sessions that focus on the feet, offering more frequent abbreviated sessions limited to the feet may be an option.

The Knee (DVD 6, 44:02 through 1:15:34)

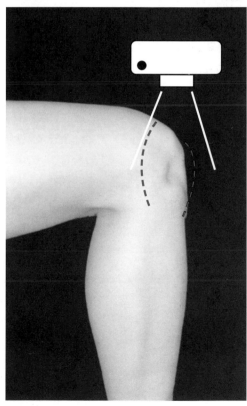

Patellar Alignment

Figure 5-13. X-ray and Photograph of Poor Patellar Tracking

This x-ray and photograph showing the angle at which the x-ray was taken beautifully demonstrate the importance of having a balance of the forces acting upon the knee and patella. The client complained of knee pain when walking down steps. This x-ray was taken from an angle above the right knee when it was bent at a similar position to that in which he experienced pain while descending steps.

It can be seen that the patella is pulled laterally by the tight tissue of the outside leg. Instead of tracking in the concave groove in the femur, it is tilted up and pulled laterally against the femoral condyle. Each time he takes a step down stairs, his patella rubs against the condyle, causing pain.

There are two basic causes of this problem. The first is the tightness and inflexibility of the lateral leg muscles and fascia, particularly the IT band and the vastus lateralis muscle. These short tissues contract when weight is placed on the bent knee, and they tilt and pull the patella laterally so that, instead of sliding in the groove of the femur, it rubs against the lateral

Figure 5-13

 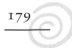

condyle each time the knee flexes. The lateral tissues must be stretched and the individual muscles must be massaged with the goals of lengthening and of separating individual compartments of different muscles so they can exert their force in the proper direction.

The second cause is the weakness of the vastus medialis muscle, which is not performing its function of pulling the patella medially so that it can track properly in the groove in the femur. Isolating and strengthening the vastus medialis, along with softening and stretching the lateral compartment will help this problem significantly.

Not all strains on joints are so easily demonstrated, but remember this photograph as an example of how weak or fibrous muscles can disrupt the proper function of joints. A knowledge of anatomy, kinesiology, and of precise Deep Tissue Massage techniques can sometimes perform wonders in treating such cases.

Soft Tissue Strategies

Many of the benefits from massage to the knee will come from helping the patella track in a straight line with the femur and tibia. If there is a problem with patellar tracking, it is most often due to excessive tightness in the lateral compartment of the upper leg. The vastus lateralis and the IT band can pull the patella laterally during knee movement as shown in the previous x-ray. The complex configuration of the adductors, abductors, hamstring, and quadriceps groups of muscles can also cause rotational forces on the deep knee joint if one group is too tight or is weak. Also, tissue build up or adhesions may form between individual muscles so that they are unable to smoothly slide past each other. In this case, several muscles may exert their force as a group rather than individually. This may alter the direction of pull through the knee. Although it is effective to clarify the separations between compartments with the fingers while the client is immobile, it is usually much more helpful to follow the division between compartments until you feel restriction and then ask the client to actively flex and extend the knee. Use this technique to separate and clarify any of the anterior, posterior, lateral, or medial muscle compartments.

Figure 5-14. Working with the Patella (DVD 6, 50:31)

Before beginning work on the patella, palpate the area to find tender and fibrous areas. Ideally, the patella should move in a proximal to distal direction without rotation during knee flexion and extension. Very lightly place your hand over the patella and ask for knee movement to test how it is tracking. Instead of moving straight up and down, does it rotate counterclockwise or clockwise? Test for lateral and medial mobility; remember that the patella can only move in these directions if the knee is fully extended. Using soft fingers, work around the patella, softening any hard areas and working with the knee in different degrees of extension. Be careful not to press the patella into the femur and tibia.

The Iliotibial Band (DVD 6, 55:39)

Almost always, work on the IT band will be beneficial for both the low back and the knees. In athletes it will usually be short, tight, and tender. The first strategy should be lengthening, followed by focused work to separate the IT band from the hamstring and quadriceps, which may be pulling it posterior or anterior.

Figure 5-15. Softening the Iliotibial Band

Work very slowly at an oblique angle from the tensor fascia latae muscle all the way down and across the knee joint. If work with the forearm is painful, use the fingertips. This is slow and meticulous work that might take fifteen minutes or more on each leg. Asking for straightening and bending of the knee will increase the effectiveness. You may want to place a pillow between the knees.

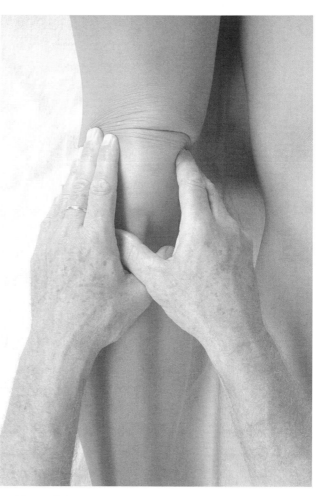

Figure 5-14

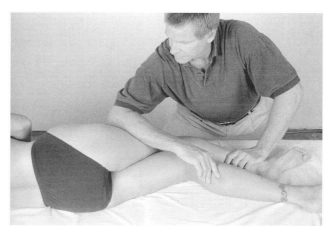

Figure 5-15

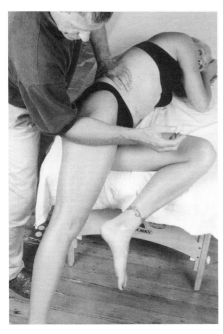

Figure 5-16

Figure 5-16. Alternative Position to Stretch the IT Band

If this position is comfortable for your client, it is an effective method of stretching the IT band while working. Have your client slide down so that her leg is hanging over the end of the table and is pulled down by gravity. The bottom leg is bent to provide stability. This can also be accomplished by having the leg hang over the side of the table, but this can impose twist on the spine.

Caution: If your client has any low back problems, this position is contraindicated.

Figure 5-17. Rolling and Lifting the IT Band

Grab the entire band and slowly roll it back and forth while visualizing lifting it from the femur.

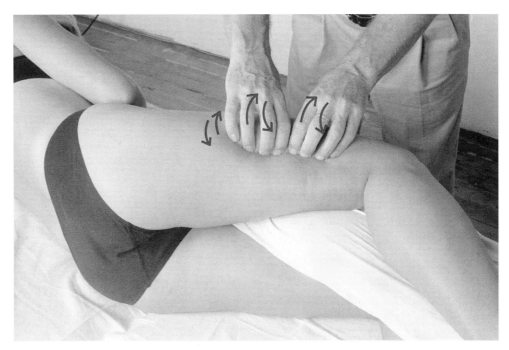

Figure 5-17

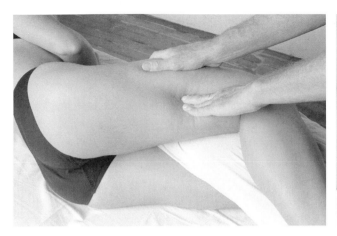

Figure 5-18a

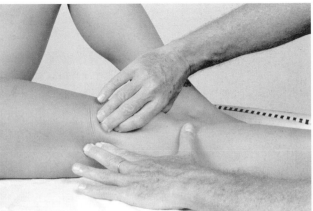

Figure 5-18b

Figures 5-18 a and b. Separating the IT Band from Adjacent Muscle Groups

This is intense work, but very beneficial. Explain to your client what you are doing and why. The major purpose of this work is to free the IT band from surrounding muscle groups so that it will not place rotational force upon the knee when these muscles contract. Using the fingers or knuckles, carefully work your way up each border to free the IT band from the adjacent muscles. Actively or passively flexing the knee joint will expedite the process and help you find adhesions that are preventing smooth movement. Imagine the compartments sliding past each other. Visualize the IT band lying between the hamstrings and quadriceps and how these muscle groups will slide alongside the IT band as they lengthen and shorten. Flexing the knee will lengthen and pull the quadriceps relative to the band, while straightening the knee will stretch the hamstrings and shorten the quadriceps.

Working with the Adductors (DVD 6, 1:04:49)
Figure 5-19. Working with the Adductors

Working the medial compartment will help create balance in the knee. Ask for slow movement, having client either bring the knee forward by flexing the hip, or extend the lower leg by straightening the knee. Clarify the separation between the individual adductor muscles, between the adductors and the hamstrings, or between the adductors and the quadriceps. Beginning with the

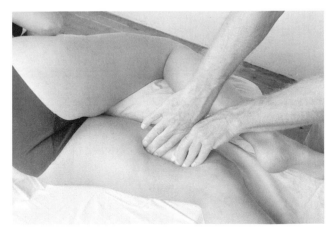

Figure 5-19

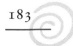

knee bent and asking for straightening of the lower leg will be most effective in separating the adductors from the hamstrings, while beginning with the knee straight and having the client flex the knee will be effective in separating the adductors from the quadriceps.

Note: The side-lying position is most effective for this work because it allows many alternatives for positioning. Both the hip and knee may be flexed or extended in any combination of positions. Notice that the upper leg is supported by a bolster.

Knee Tracking
Figure 5-20. Tracking the Patella

The quadriceps are probably the most important muscles to work with when there are complaints of knee pain. Often, if you ask the client to raise the knee, you will feel the patella rotate or pull to one side. You may also feel the whole quadriceps contract unevenly due to tightness. This can cause torsion in the deep knee joint or disrupt the movement of the patella over the femur. Initially, broad forearm strokes with the client lying passively are effective in softening tight quadriceps. After initial broad softening work, place fingers or knuckles on either side of knee for separating different quadriceps compartments and ask the client to lift the knee by sliding the foot towards the buttocks. If you feel uneven torsion, apply pressure in order to force the knee to track straight.

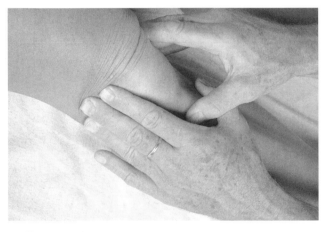

Figure 5-20

Figure 5-21. Seated Active Knee Movement Strategy

With the client sitting on the edge of the table, anchor in areas of pain or restriction with your fingers and ask for extension of the knee. In more severe cases, stop movement short of full extension to decrease chance of inflammation, which may result from pressure on the patella.

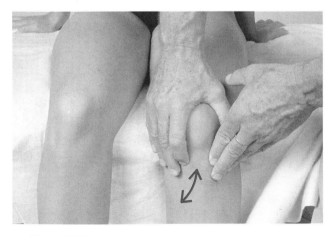

Figure 5-21

Figure 5-22. Working the Knee with Maximum Flexion

Flexing the hip allows for many possibilities of stretch and rotation to the knee while working with the soft tissues around the knee. Stretch will be localized at the knee rather than at the upper quadriceps and the therapist's other hand can rotate the tibia in relation to the femur.

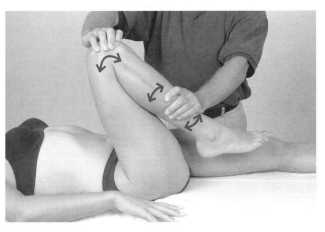

Figure 5-22

Figure 5-23. Posterior Knee Work

Work carefully behind the knee if you feel the need to address the tendons of the gastrocnemius or hamstrings. Have the knee slightly flexed in order to soften the area and allow for easy access. The popliteus and plantaris muscles, although not crucial for knee function, may be tight or inflamed. Gentle work to soften and lengthen these muscles may help resolve posterior knee pain. Work slowly with very soft fingers. Often pain in the posterior region is due to swelling in the synovial capsule of the knee rather than tight muscles, and will not respond well to work. It is also very effective to flex the knee, anchor the hamstrings, and then straighten the leg to stretch the hamstrings. Remember that the gastrocnemius crosses the knee joint and may impact knee function. Check to see if one head of the gastrocnemius is tighter than the other and creating strain, and if so, work on it.

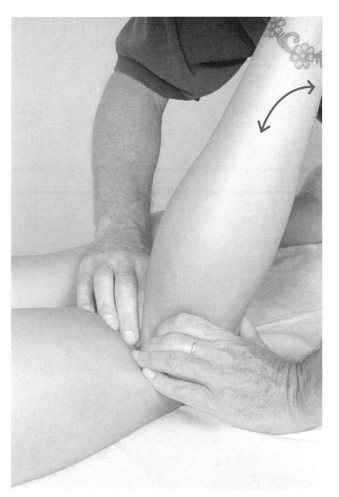

Figure 5-23

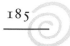

Strengthening Strategies (DVD 6, 1:08:53)

Pain in a joint will usually have the effect of sending inhibitory nerve responses to the muscles, which results in atrophy and weakness. This weakness is one reason why a minor acute injury will sometimes turn into a chronic inflammation. Simple exercises that take only five or ten minutes a day can have profound effects on alleviating knee pain.

Pain in the knee may come from lack of stability and imbalances in strength between different muscles associated with stabilizing the knee joint and patella. Ninety percent of the clients I see for knee pain have had dramatic improvement doing strengthening and flexibility exercises, while soft tissue work by itself, although very helpful, has not been as effective.

In the early stages of strengthening, an inflamed joint may not tolerate movement until the inflammation has decreased. The safest strategy is to progress from isometric strengthening exercises that keep the knee joint immobile, to more complex exercises involving flexion and extension of the joint.

Figure 5-24. Isometric Knee Strengthening (DVD 6, 1:10:17)

For acute pain, the first step might be simple isometric contractions of the quadriceps with the knee straightened to a few degrees short of full extension. Place a rolled towel under the knee and have your client push the knee straight down into the towel while concentrating on contracting the quadriceps muscles.

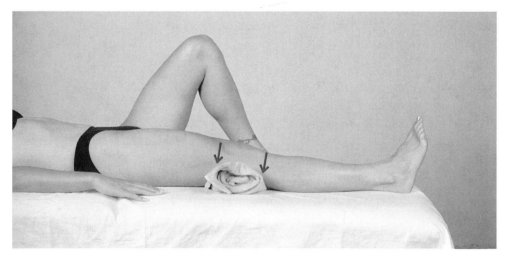

Figure 5-24

Figures 5-25 a and b. Straight Leg Raises for Quadriceps Strengthening (6 1:12:20)

The straight leg lift is the most effective of the simple strengthening exercises. It focuses on the rectus femoris muscle, which is also a hip flexor, but also strengthens all of the quadriceps group. It is very important to have the knee fully extended to allow a full contraction of the vastus medialis, which stabilizes patella glide. Ankle weights ranging from one to twelve pounds should be used, building up to three sets of ten repetitions. When three sets become easy, increase weight.

Movement should be slow with a few seconds of holding at the top and bottom. Notice that the other knee is bent to protect and support the lower back. Placing a folded towel under the lower back will further support the lumbars.

After your client can tolerate straight leg strengthening that prevents knee joint movement, it is beneficial to add more complex exercises that strengthen the joint through a range of motion that more closely approximates normal stresses upon the knee.

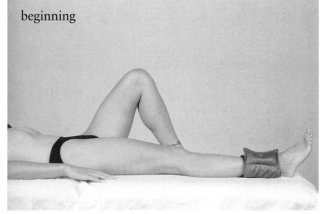

beginning

Figure 5-25a

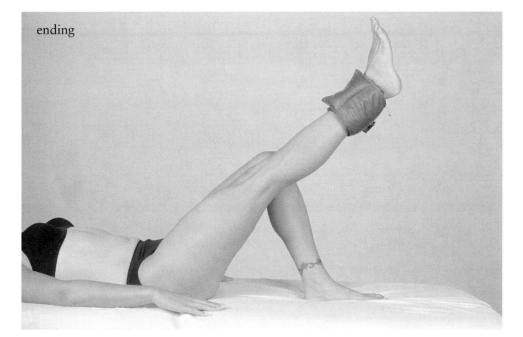

ending

Figure 5-25b

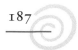

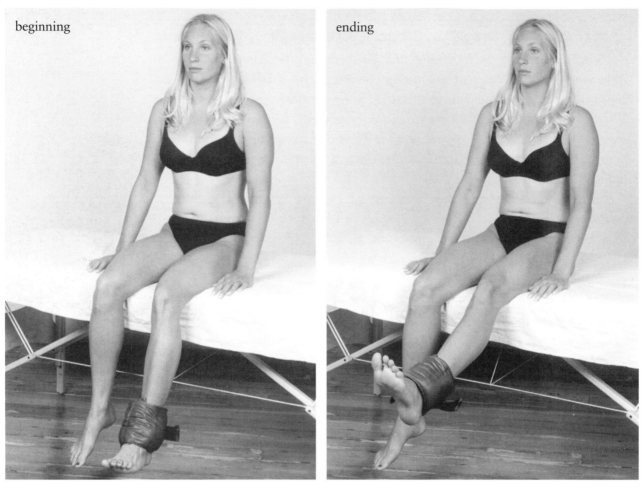

beginning

ending

Figure 5-26a   **Figure 5-26b**

Figures 5-26 a and b. Leg Extensions for Quadriceps Strengthening (DVD 6, 1:15:34)

Begin with the knee bent less than ninety degrees (beginning) and extend the knee to approximately five degrees short of full extension (ending). Exercises limiting the range of flexion and extension are called "short arc quad sets." Stopping the extension a few degrees short of straight prevents the patella from being compressed against the femur by the contraction of the quadriceps. These exercises can be performed with ankle weights or with Nautilus or free-weight leg extension machines at a gym. Progress weight as tolerated.

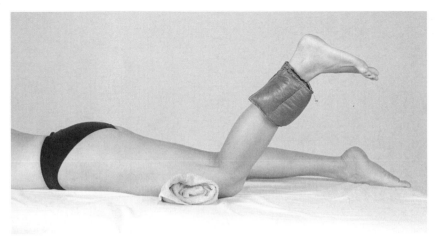

Figure 5-27a

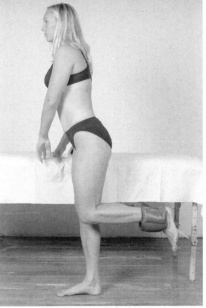

Figures 5-27 a and b. Hamstring Curl Alternatives

Both these exercises begin with the knee straight and move to flex-ion of ninety degrees. Use ankle weights from one to ten pounds working up to three sets of ten repetitions Notice that in the prone position, you may put a pillow just above the joint to minimize pressure on the patella.

For most people, work with the quadriceps and hamstrings is sufficient. If the client is ambitious, it may be helpful to strengthen all aspects of the knee. If desired, the following exercises may be added after a week or two.

Figure 5-27b

Figures 5-28 a and b. Adductor Strengthening Alternatives

Often, no weights are needed. Position the upper leg forward in whichever position is most comfortable; for people with low back symptoms, placing the upper knee on a pillow, flexed forward puts less stress on the low back. Raise the bottom leg sixteen to twenty inches off the table. As with all exercises shown, complete three sets of ten repetitions.

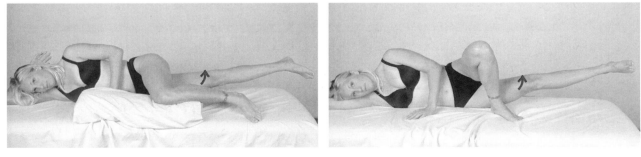

Figure 5-28a   Figure 5-28b

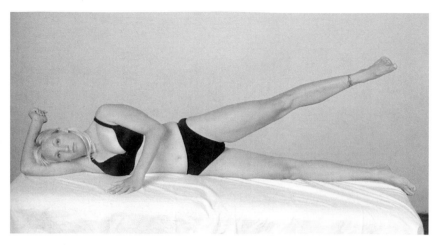

Figure 5-29

Figure 5-29. Abductor Strengthening

The bottom knee may be bent forward to provide stability.

Stretching Strategies

Figures 5-30 a and b. Quadriceps Stretching Alternatives

Pull the ankle towards the gluteals and hold for forty-five seconds. Use the hand on the same side of the leg being worked. The farther back the hip is extended, the more stretch on the rectus fermoris.

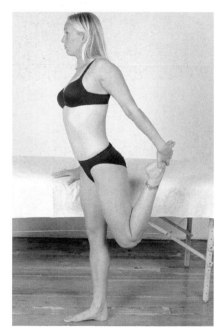

Figure 5-30a

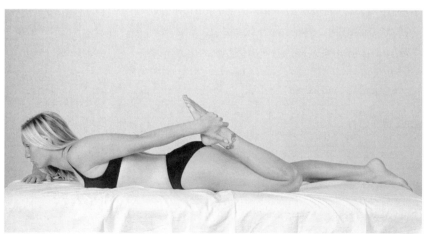

Figure 5-30b

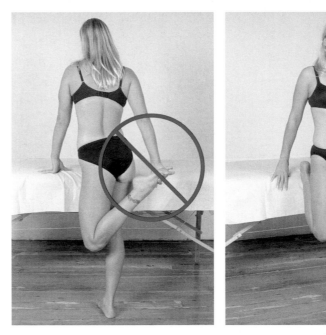

Figure 5-31

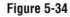

Figure 5-32

Figure 5-31. Improper Quadriceps Stretching

Stretching using the opposite hand places strain in the knee and low back.

Figure 5-32. Quadriceps Stretch for Secure Balance

This stretch is effective for clients who have difficulty grabbing their ankle or with balance.

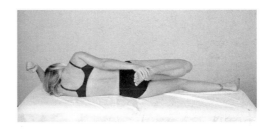

Figure 5-33

Figure 5-33. Side-Lying Quadriceps Stretch

Side-lying is an effective method of stretching the quadriceps in nonweight bearing while extending the hip to enable greater stretch.

Figure 5-34. Supine Hamstring Stretch

This position is safer for the back than many of the standing hamstring stretches. Have clients be sure that the knee is fully extended rather than bent. Placing the strap over the front of the foot to dorsiflex the ankle will also stretch the gastrocnemius, while placing the strap back by the heel or grabbing the lower leg just distal to the knee will isolate the hamstring.

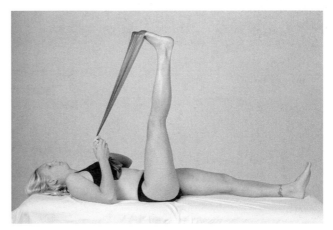

Figure 5-34

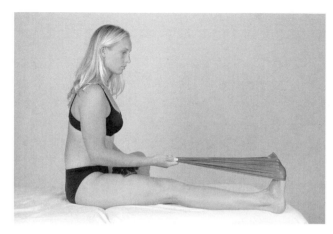

Figure 5-35

Figure 5-35. Seated Hamstring Stretch

This stretch is as effective as that in the previous example, but may cause back strain. Advise clients to be sure to keep the back straight rather than flexing forward.

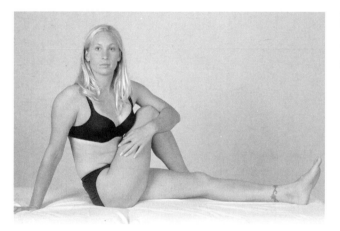

Figure 5-36

Figure 5-36. Iliotibial Band Stretch

Keeping the back straight, pull the knee towards the opposite side.

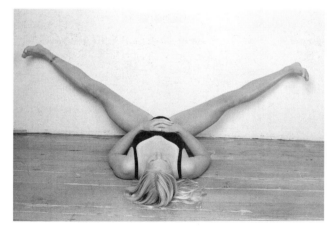

Figure 5-37

Figure 5-37. Adductor Stretch

This stretch is performed lying on back with the buttocks against the wall and letting gravity pull the legs apart. This stretch may also be done in a seated upright position, but will place more strain on the back.

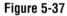

Tennis Elbow and Golfer's Elbow (DVD 7, 52:47 through 1:00:12)

Tennis elbow (lateral epicondylitis) and golfer's elbow (medial epicondylitis) are basically a tendonitis of either the outside or inside of the elbow. Don't be fooled by their athletic nomenclature; they are a common problem with the general population and can be very debilitating. Knowing how to treat these conditions will add to the success of your practice. They are usually related to tight and weak muscles in either the extensor compartment of the forearm (tennis elbow) or the flexor compartment (golfer's elbow). Symptoms often appear suddenly after performance of an unaccustomed activity that involves use of the forearm muscles, such as scrubbing floors or pruning hedges. In the early stages symptoms will often disappear with a few treatments without strengthening or flexibility exercises. If the problem is chronic, the healing process is considerably longer and will be enhanced by client participation in home stretching, strengthening, and anti-inflammatory routines.

Soft Tissue Strategies

Figure 5-38. Tennis Elbow Strategies

A tight and inflexible supinator muscle is the primary culprit in tennis elbow, but softening all of the arm muscles, including the lower triceps, is beneficial. In severe cases, pain at the lateral epicondyle of the elbow can be so extreme that it prevents everyday activities such as brushing teeth or grasping a pencil. Softening the entire wrist extensor compartment, including the belly of the muscles, is important. The therapist can manipulate the wrist into pronation or supination and flexion or extension to focus stretch on specific muscles. Work on the point of tenderness with cross-fiber strokes and explain that it may be a bit sore for a day or two. Do not try to accomplish too much at one time; frequently spaced multiple sessions are safer and more beneficial. Notice that the wrist is flexed and pronated to place supinator and the extensor muscles on a stretch. Asking the client to lift the wrist against your resistance will help deter-

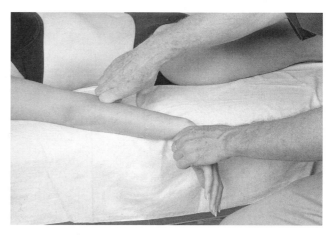

Figure 5-38

mine where localized strain patterns exist. In addition to the kneading work of regular massage, remember to stretch the tissue rather than simply rolling over it. Spend time separating muscle compartments with your fingers and do some work above the elbow to decompress the joint.

Explain the importance of a consistent stretching and strengthening program, refraining from any activity that causes pain, and use frequent applications of ice.

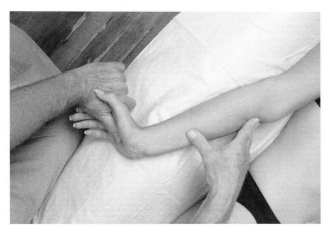

Figure 5-39. Golfer's Elbow Strategies

Work in the same manner as with tennis elbow but on the flexor compartment of the arm. Notice that the wrist is now extended and supinated to place the flexors and pronator teres into a stretch.

Figure 5-39

Strengthening Strategies

Figures 5-40 a. Forearm Flexor Strengthening—Palm Up; and b. Forearm Extensor Strengthening—Palm Down

Using either flexible tubing or small weights, have client flex the wrist or extend the wrist. She should begin with very little resistance and only five repetitions to determine if the wrist is strong enough to tolerate strengthening. Often, if there is a flare up, it will not occur until the next day, so clients should be conservative in increasing resistance.

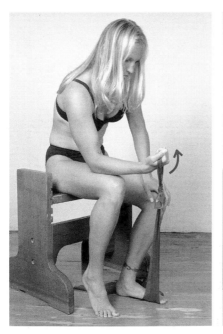

Figure 5-40a

Figure 5-40b

Stretching Strategies

Figures 5-41a. Stretching Forearm Extensors—Palm Down; and b. Stretching Forearm Flexors—Palm Up

The elbow is completely extended and the wrist is bent and hand pulled down toward the body, palm facing in for the first, or palm facing out for the second. These stretches should be held for thirty seconds. Clients should not overstretch, but repeat the movements frequently during the day.

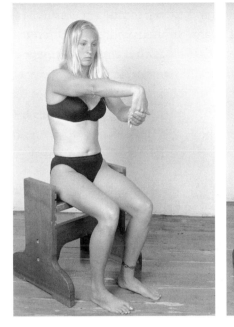

Figure 5-41a　　　　**Figure 5-41b**

Carpal Tunnel Syndrome

SOFT TISSUE WORK FOR CARPAL TUNNEL is similar to treatment of tennis elbow, but is more complicated because it involves nerve compression or entrapment. First, it is important to have a medical diagnosis to ensure that the symptoms are actually carpal tunnel syndrome rather than tendonitis. This is a serious and complicated condition; beware of workshops that promise a "cure" for carpal tunnel with a few secret strokes. You will not be doing your client a favor if you slightly improve symptoms so that he can return with a false sense of safety to the same activity that caused the symptoms. Even with excellent treatment, carpal tunnel syndrome rarely resolves without addressing the original causes of the problem. Tennis elbow can occur after one incident that strains the elbow, but carpal tunnel is almost always an overuse injury involving repetitive strain on the wrist. The condition is further complicated by the fact that the symptoms can also be a result of tightness in the anterior neck and chest, or impingement of the nerves at the thoracic outlet. A nerve conduction test, administered by a neurologist, is the most accurate method to determine where the nerves are impinged or damaged.

This is not to say that Deep Tissue Massage is not a very effective tool in treating carpal tunnel syndrome. Often it is the missing link in conventional treatment that leads to a cure. Treatment should cover area from the clavicle and scalenes, down the arm past the wrist to the palm of the hand. Review the section on working with the scalenes for thoracic outlet strategies (Figures 3-104–107). Continue down the arm, paying particular attention to the triceps just above the elbow. Give slow, meticulous work to both the flexor and extensor compartments of the forearm, and then proceed to the wrist and hand.

Figure 5-42. Working around the Carpal Tunnel

The goal should be to decompress and soften tissue around the wrist. Detailed work anywhere around the wrist is helpful and rarely causes a flare up. Be careful not to compress the median nerves by working where they pass through the carpal tunnel, and have your client alert you if any work your are performing elicits symptoms associated with carpal tunnel syndrome: numbness, tingling, any sign that the nerve, rather than the tissue, is being worked on. Work to open and widen the carpal tunnel and to stretch tissue in the palm.

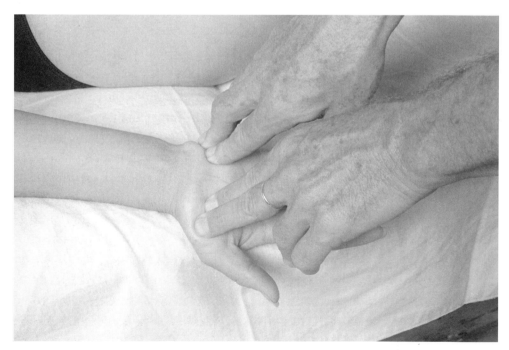

Figure 5-42

The Low Back (DVD 6, 1:31:49)

FOR THE NORMAL REACTIONS OF LOW BACK STIFFNESS and slight pain that occasionally occur as a result of strenuous activity, massage is probably the most effective treatment available. Often, more serious symptoms of low back pain also respond extremely well to massage, but the problem is that "one person's medicine is another person's poison." It is extremely important that your goal be to *improve* symptoms, not *cure* them. Do not overwork a painful area, and try to not place too much pressure on yourself by having expectations that are too high.

There are no hard and fast rules for treating the various complaints associated with back pain, including sciatica. The safest policy is to do general work around the low back and pelvis just as you would in a normal massage, taking particular care to have your client lying in a *neutral* (pain free) position. You may need to use extra pillows as props and to have client change positions frequently so that areas do not stiffen from being immobile for too long a time. Working on the quadratus lumborum, the rotators, IT band, and psoas muscles, as demonstrated in previous sections, all may be effective strategies.

Although the majority of people report improvement and can be very grateful to you, be prepared for a certain small percentage to report increased symptoms that manifest themselves several hours after the massage or the next day. This does not necessarily mean that you have done something wrong. The symptoms may be attributable to other causes besides the massage. If you have been careful and not placed strain on the back, almost always, the increased symptoms will subside in a day or two, and improvement will result. It is important to prepare the client for the possibility so that she will not be alarmed. Ask your client to call you and report how she is feeling.

Because of the complicated nature of the back and the sacroiliac joint, and their associated symptoms, only the most basic and safe techniques will be mentioned here. Often, five minutes of simple instructions about pelvic stabilization and proper posture will do more good than hours of manual work. It is well worth your time to try to determine what is the cause of the problem rather than spending hours trying to release a spasm which will return the next time the client bends over or sits in a poorly designed chair. Note the instructions on how to get up from the seated position in Chapter Four.

Soft Tissue Strategies

Pain in the lower back frequently manifests itself in spasmed muscles. Releasing these muscles will often bring significant relief in varying degrees, but the trade-off is that the increased flexibility may result in less stability in the joints. Striking a balance between these two extremes is the elusive key to successful work. The exercises that follow in the next section may prove to be the answer to providing a balance between flexibility and stability so the client may remain pain free.

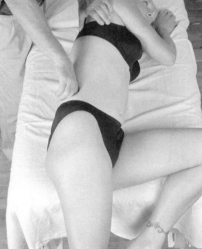

Figure 5-43

Figure 5-43. Stretching the Quadratus Lumborum While Working

Work the quadratus the same way you would in a regular massage, being careful to not apply too much broad pressure because of the floating ribs and the proximity of the kidneys. Use the fingers or knuckles and focus on the origin and insertion in addition to the belly of the muscle. One key to quadratus work is to determine if one side is tighter than the other, and work for balance between the two sides. It may be that only one side is tight, and that work on the relaxed side will be unproductive or even exacerbate symptoms. Never just "dive in" without having a purpose to your work.

Notice that in this example the client's left leg is hanging over the table. This will afford a greater stretch to the quadratus but is not advised for a person with an acute, severe flare-up.

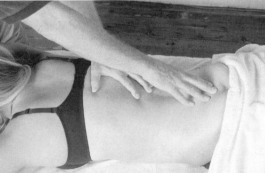

Figure 5-44

Figure 5-44. Working with the Sacrum

Gentle work around the sacrum is often useful and always feels good. Frequently, the sacrum will be immobilized at the first sign of lower back pain. Freeing soft tissue restrictions to enable more freedom of movement is often helpful. Utilize the side-lying position if your client is uncomfortable in the prone position or place a pillow under the abdomen.

Precautions: Be sure to apply oblique pressure and to move slowly.

Working the Low Back in Flexion and Extension (DVD 7, 0:22)

One of the keys to a healthy low back is the maintenance of a neutral position for the pelvis both in sitting and in standing. If the pelvis tilts too far forward, the lumbar spine can be driven too far into extension or "sway back." If the pelvis is tucked under, the lumbar spine may be forced into a flat or forward flexed position. People who have too much extension in the low back often have difficulty bending forward into flexion, while those who have a flat lumbar spine often complain of pain in extension or back bending.

Deep Tissue Massage can be very helpful in softening and stretching the muscles that restrict the ability of the low back and spine to move through the full range of motion from flexion to extension. The goal of the therapist should be to enable a greater range of motion in the restricted direction by working on the back in a position that will stretch tight muscles. For a client with an extreme lordosis and limited flexion, your work will be most productive if you place her into a position of comfortable flexion to stretch the lumbar fascia and muscles so that the pelvis can begin to move into a less anterior tilt.

For a client who has difficulty back bending, the strategy would be to place her as far into a position of extension as is comfortable to work. In both cases, as the muscles relax and the range of motion increases, you can incrementally extend the positions to increase the stretch.

In attempting to work with the pelvis in positions of either spinal extension or flexion, the prone position limits your options for manipulating the angle of pelvic tilt. Although it is possible to enable small deviations in the pelvic angle by the use of pillows under the abdomen, you are basically limited to a neutral position. The side-lying position offers the advantages of working in either neutral, flexion, or extension while applying substantial force without the hazard of driving the lumbar vertebrae too anterior. Ask for active movement from anterior to posterior tilt on the pelvis to help break spasm patterns and extend range of motion.

◎ Caution: In the condition known as spondylolisthesis, placing your client into a position of back extension is contraindicated. In this condition, one vertebra has already slipped too far anterior, and movement into spinal extension could seriously exacerbate the situation. It would be very unusual for a client to be unaware that she has this condition. The pain associated with spondy-

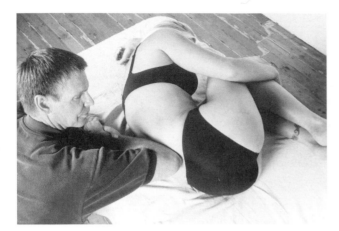

Figure 5-45

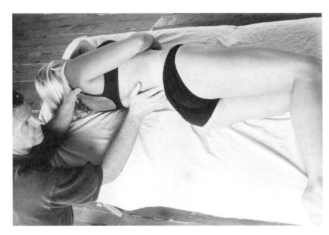

Figure 5-46

lolisthesis would normally necessitate medical evaluation and a proper diagnosis, and you would expect that your client would inform you of the condition. If your client informs you that she has spondylolisthesis, be careful to keep the spine in a neutral or slightly flexed posture while working.

Figure 5-45. Working the Low Back in Flexion

Have your client bring the knees forward or lie in the fetal position. This will stretch tight lumbar fascia and low back muscles. Work in an upward and downward direction away from the iliac crest with the goal of increasing mobility in the lumbars and pelvis and softening the lumbar fascia.

Figure 5-46. Working the Low Back in Extension

Bring the knees back so that there is an increase in the lumbar curve in the opposite direction from the fetal position. Ask for feedback from your client to assure that she is always comfortable. Work incrementally to increase more mobility and ease in extension by occasionally moving the legs back to slightly increase the pelvic tilt.

Strengthening Strategies

These exercises are designed to address chronic low level back pain and for back maintenance. They should not be suggested in the early stages of an acute episode. Keep any exercises simple and add new variations one at a time so that if flare-ups occur, it is possible to determine the cause. If pain increases either during or after these exercises, have clients discontinue them for the time being. It does not necessarily mean that this is the wrong exercise; it may be that the inflammation is still too great and must first be resolved before strengthening is increased. The following exercises should be performed on a firm surface, not on a bed. Consider referring your client to a physical therapist who specializes in pelvic stabilization training or to a Pilates trainer. Both of these have extensive training and experience in the nuances of strengthening to determine which exercises are best for each individual.

A simple pelvic tilt is the safest exercise to begin with. Simply have the client lie in supine position with her feet on the table and both knees bent, similar to the starting position for abdominal "crunches." Have your client slowly push the lower back to the table and hold for ten seconds. If your client has a pronounced lordosis or sway back, placing a folded towel under the lumbars will help maintain a neutral posture. Move from this to actively tucking the pelvis under. Ask clients to hold the posture for ten or more seconds.

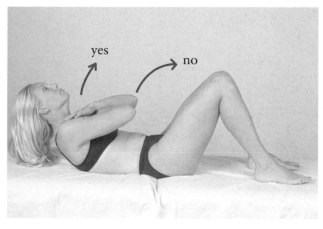

Figure 5-47

Figure 5-47. Abdominal Strengthening

Straight crunches are probably the most effective and safest exercise. Have your client lift the head and chest up towards the ceiling in the direction of the arrows in the photograph. Ask her not to try to roll forward or "curl" up towards the knees but to move slowly and only go as far as is comfortable. Crossing the arms over the chest prevents using the shoulder girdle to help in lifting the torso. Build up to fifteen repetitions.

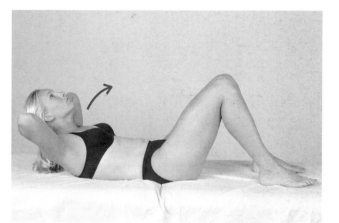

Figure 5-48

Figure 5-48. Abdominal Strengthening—Neck Supported

If the client has neck pain, supporting the head with the arms removes strain from the neck.

Figure 5-49. Abdominal Strengthening—Lower Abdomen

Resting the legs on a chair or table isolates the lower abdomen.

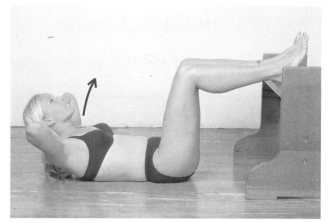

Figure 5-49

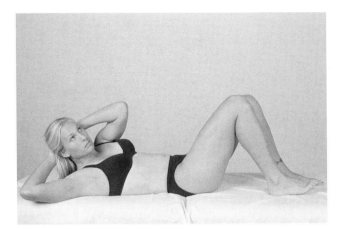

Figure 5-50a

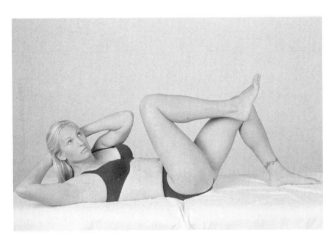

Figure 5-50b

Figures 5-50 a and b. Isolating the Obliques

Lifting the left elbow across toward the right knee will strengthen the obliques. In more advanced stages, the knee can be brought up to meet the elbow.

Figure 5-51. Stability and Balance Exercise

Clients sometimes complain that chiropractic adjustments don't last. Strengthening the small vertebral muscles is often helpful. This exercise not only strengthens the large muscle groups such as the hamstrings, gluteals, and erectors, but also the small muscles such as the rotatores, which stabilize individual vertebrae. Have client hold the opposite arm and leg up for five seconds, then bring the arm and leg down and repeat five to ten times before switching to the other side.

Figure 5-52. Gluteal and Hamstring Strengthening

Have client slowly lift one leg at a time and repeat five to fifteen times.

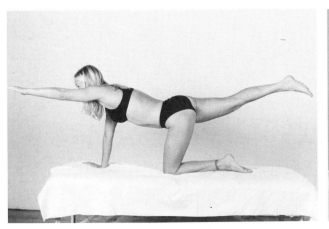

Figure 5-51

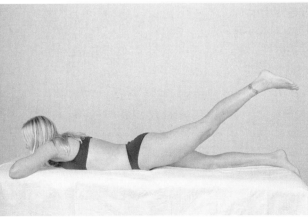

Figure 5-52

Stretching Strategies

Figure 5-53. Rotator Stretch

Have one ankle resting on the other knee with the leg turned out as much as possible. Reach through the rotated leg to grab behind the other knee and then pull it towards the body. If comfortable, client may pull the knee from the front rather than from behind. Hold for forty-five seconds and then switch legs.

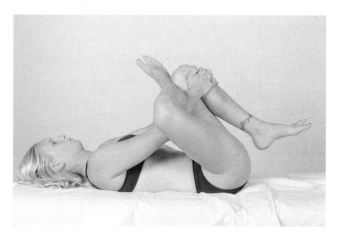

Figure 5-53

Figure 5-54. Low Back Stretch

Have client pull both knees towards chest and hold for thirty seconds and repeat several times a day. Most people feel good performing this stretch, but a few report increased symptoms because of the movement of the lumbars into flexion. If comfortable, a person can progress to pulling one leg at a time while the other leg is extended.

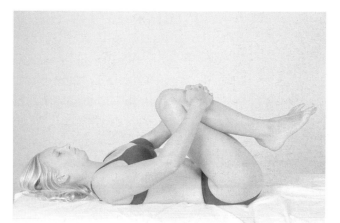

Figure 5-54

Figure 5-55. Back Extension Stretch

Low back strain is often a result of the lumbars being too posterior, or too little lumbar lordosis. Sometimes clients are hesitant to try this stretch because of pain if they bend too far backwards. It is very important for them only to stretch as far as is comfortable and then, over a period of days or weeks, extend that threshold point so they have greater mobility. Gently moving into extension and holding for forty-five seconds can give relief to many people and occasionally effect a miraculous improvement. The client will usually know immediately if this exercise is helpful. If so, it may be repeated many times every day. This is a flexibility stretch, not a strengthening stretch, so they should use the upper body and arms to lift and hold this position rather than attempting to lift with the low back.

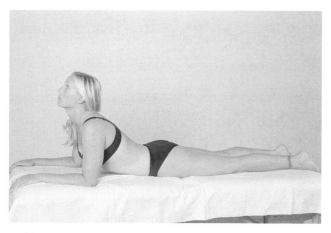

Figure 5-55

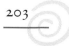

Sciatica (DVD 6, 1:21:57)

If the sciatic nerve is impinged, it can send many different sensations down the hamstrings and leg, sometimes all the way to the foot. Most often, these symptoms of spasm, pain, or numbness occur unilaterally, but they may affect both legs. Deep Tissue Massage will usually improve symptoms, at least temporarily, by relaxing the muscle spasms, which are caused by the inflamed nerve. For lasting relief, the mechanical problems that are impinging the nerve must be addressed. If possible, your client should see an expert such as an osteopath, chiropractor, or physical therapist to determine where the nerve is being impinged. If the cause is a misaligned vertebra or disc, massage to the low back may be contraindicated because it could exacerbate the problem. (For impingement of the nerve by tight muscles in the pelvis, see the next section: "Piriformis Syndrome.")

Of course, tight muscles can be exerting compressive or rotational forces upon the bones or disc. Sometimes massage can decompress and restore balance in the lumbar area and significantly help sciatica. The difficulty for a massage therapist is that few of us have the training to accurately assess exactly how to work to decompress the nerve near the spine. When working on a client who has been diagnosed with sciatica, be careful to keep the spine in a neutral and comfortable position. To minimize the amount of pressure on the spine, work with fingers rather than with a broad surface such as the forearm, and have your client keep you apprised of any increase in symptoms.

Soft Tissue Strategies

Creating balance and ease in the lumbar region should be your goal. Decompress the area by softening the lumbar fascia and the quadratus lumborum as demonstrated in earlier sections. Notice if there are rotational forces on the spine caused by tight muscles: Is the quadratus in spasm on one side, which causes a side-bending of the spine? Are the psoas muscles causing anterior strain on the lumbars because they are both tight, or is the psoas tight unilaterally and causing rotational strain? Are the gluteus medius and minimus causing strain in the pelvis? Work for balance between the front and back and between the left and right sides.

After creating balance in the lumbar region and pelvis, work down the leg wherever sciatic tightness is present. Remember that the nerve can be impinged at more than one place.

Strengthening and Stretching Strategies

Most of the strengthening and stretching exercises that are listed in the section for low back pain are applicable for sciatica. For severe cases, it is best to refer to an expert.

Piriformis Syndrome and Sciatica

Sometimes the sciatic nerve is compressed by tight muscles in the pelvis instead of at its exit from the spinal cord. This condition is labeled *Piriformis Syndrome* because a tight piriformis is often the cause. The sciatic nerve can actually run superficial to, deep to, or even through the piriformis, depending on the individual. Patient and meticulous work on all the rotators is needed. Keep a global view of the problem, remembering that the piriformis may be tight because motor nerves from the spine are making it contract. Work for creating ease in the low back and do not restrict your work to the piriformis.

◎ LOCATING THE PIRIFORMIS

Some students have felt intimidated by trying to precisely locate rotators, and particularly the piriformis. First, study the anatomy drawing showing the rotators (Figure 3-36), and also note the sciatic nerve as it descends below the piriformis. Locate the top of the trochanter. This is the insertion of the piriformis tendon, but it will be easier to palpate the tendon approximately one-half inch medial to the trochanter. Now find the halfway point along the lateral border of the sacrum. (If you are unsure of where the lateral border is, just put one finger on the top of the sacrum below the fifth lumbar vertebra and another finger at the bottom of the sacrum, right above the coccyx and then visualize a point midway between these points.) If you were to draw a line between the top of the trochanter and the midpoint of either the sacrum or its lateral border, the piriformis would follow that line directly below the gluteus maximus.

It is not crucial to know the names of all the rotators, as long as you can determine where tightness is. But while you are looking at the drawing, why not take some time to study and memorize the different muscles? It will help you understand the complexity of the forces acting upon the pelvis.

Soft Tissue Strategies for the Piriformis

Softening and stretching the piriformis (as shown in Figures 3-38 and 3-39) can be extremely effective in reducing or even curing sciatica. The primary difference between the usual deep tissue approaches to the rotators and working with piriformis syndrome is that more care must be taken not to further irritate an already inflamed sciatic nerve. Ask your client to inform you of any nerve sensations that travel down the leg and alter either your pressure or the direction of force accordingly. Remember always to work obliquely and never to press directly into the pelvis. Be sure to work the piriformis at its tendinous attachment at the trochanter.

Be careful not to go in too aggressively in attempting to work through the gluteus maximus in order to contact the rotators. I have seen numerous clients who had deep bruises from overzealous work in this area. Review the section on palpation in Chapter One and visualize sinking through the gluteus and directing your attention to the piriformis. You should be able to feel the tight rotators running beneath the gluteus approximately in a perpendicular direction.

The Shoulder (DVD 7, 19:04)

MANY SHOULDER INJURIES are due to strains to the rotator cuff and concomitant weakness, which interferes with the intricate functions of the joint. As pain increases, major muscles often shorten to splint against excess movement of the joint. This, in turn, may compress the shoulder. Although very helpful, massage by itself, cannot always cure a shoulder problem or frozen shoulder. A combination of soft tissue release, strengthening, and flexibility exercises is the most effective strategy. I have had many clients express their gratitude for giving them the self-reliance to cure long-standing shoulder problems by performing a few simple exercises at home.

Soft Tissue Strategies

Use many of the same techniques that you would use in general massage, but work specifically with individual rotator cuff muscles and work more slowly. Test for limitations to internal or external shoulder rotation as demonstrated in the section on general shoulder girdle strategies.

Figure 5-56. Supine Shoulder Girdle Work

Distracting (tractioning) the shoulder joint should be a major goal to relieve compression of the humerus in the glenoid fossa. While gently pulling on the humerus, massage any painful or tight areas. At the same time, you may internally or externally rotate the humerus. Clarify the different muscle compartments with precise and meticulous attention or broader strokes. Working with the pectoralis major is shown here. Similar work may be performed with the deltoid, trapezius, the teres major, and minor and the scapula itself as shown in previous sections.

Figure 5-57. Prone Shoulder Girdle Work With Distraction and Rotation of Humerus (DVD 7, 29:12)

Move the arm into positions of internal or external rotation, and into positions of abduction to stretch the various muscles of the rotator cuff. Move the arm to a position of restriction and then work areas of tightness. Then, try to extend the range of motion a bit further and continue working. Notice use of the therapist's arm to provide movement leverage for rotation of the humerus.

Strengthening Strategies (DVD 7, 45:20)

With shoulder injuries, often the small muscles "shut down" and let the larger muscles such as the trapezius and deltoid do the work. It is necessary to retrain these muscles using light weights so that the major muscles are not used instead.

◎ In addition to strengthening the smaller muscles, it is often helpful to "detrain" the large muscles such as the upper trapezius. Have your client raise her arm from the side, up to shoulder level, and notice that almost always the sore shoulder

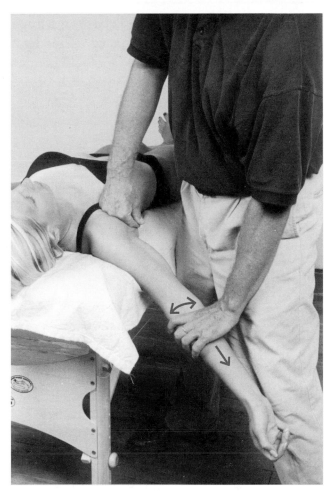

Figure 5-56

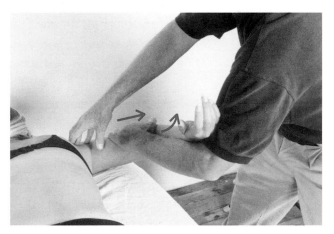

Figure 5-57

will be lifted by the trapezius. Teach the ability to raise the arm keeping the shoulders depressed by not using the trapezius. Detraining the trapezius will help to regain proper movement patterns and recruit the smaller muscles.

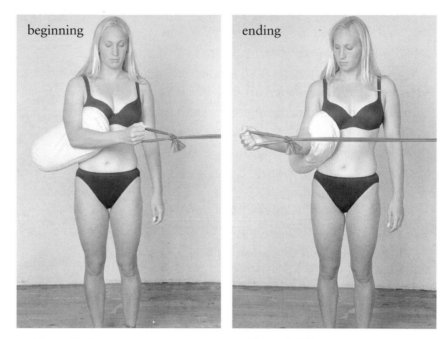

beginning

ending

Figure 5-58a   **Figure 5-58b**

Figures 5-58 a and b. Rotator Cuff Strengthening—External Rotation

Have client begin with arm reaching across abdomen in a position of internal rotation and slowly pull the elastic tubing across the body as far as is comfortable. She should take care that the only rotational movement is with the humerus rather than turning the whole body. Having the client hold a towel or small pillow against the hip will insure that the elbow stays in the proper position.

Strengthening internal rotation is less important than external rotation, but if the client is not overdeveloped in the chest, it may help. Client should begin with arm externally rotated and slowly move towards internal rotation—just the opposite from the previous exercise. Make sure that only the arm is performing the movement.

Figures 5-59 a and b. Supraspinatus Strengthening

Have your client slowly lift the arm to shoulder level at a forty-five degree angle from the body, taking care to insure that the upper trapezius is not overworking. Use a light weight such as a can of soup so that the major muscles will not be recruited. The arm should only be lifted to horizontal; any movement above that will only be accomplished by rotation of the scapula rather than the muscles you are attempting to strengthen. If this exercise causes pain, try holding the can with the thumb pointed upwards. Work up to two sets of ten repetitions.

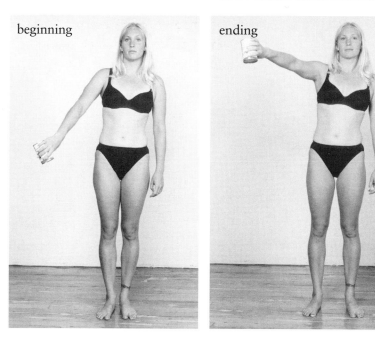

beginning

ending

Figure 5-59a

Figure 5-59b

Figures 5-60 a and b. Infraspinatus Strengthening

While lying in prone position at the edge of the table, have your client raise the affected arm to horizontal at a right angle to the body. Often no weight will be necessary. Two sets of ten repetitions should be sufficient. Having your client try the exercise on the uninvolved shoulder will often be helpful to demonstrate how much weaker the sore shoulder is and the need for strengthening exercises.

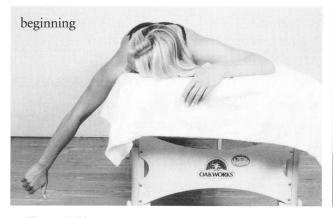

beginning

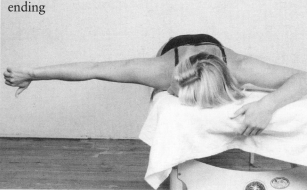

ending

Figure 5-60a

Figure 5-60b

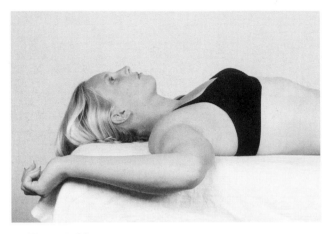

Figure 5-61

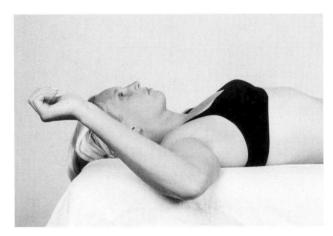

Figure 5-62

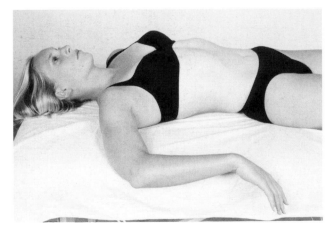

Figure 5-63

Determining Restrictions in Arm Rotation

In order to determine which stretches will be effective, it is important to determine where shoulder rotation is limited. When there is shoulder pain, almost always internal and/or external rotation will be limited. Stretching and decompressing the joint are very important goals, but it is crucial to be patient and not stretch too aggressively.

In order to determine if the client is limited in either internal or external rotation of the arm it is helpful to abduct the arm to shoulder level while the client is in supine position. Flex the elbow to ninety degrees and rotate the humerus internally and externally. Notice if one shoulder is more limited than the other. If the arm is limited in internal rotation, then more time needs to be spent on softening and lengthening the external rotators, which are located in the posterior shoulder/rotator cuff area. Conversely, if the shoulder is limited in external rotation, then work will be most beneficial on the internal rotators.

Figure 5-61. Ideal External Rotation of the Humerus
Arm should rest easily on the table.

Figure 5-62. Limited External Rotation of the Humerus
Note inability of the arm to rotate externally toward horizontal. Concentrate work on the anterior shoulder muscles.

Figure 5-63. Ideal Internal Rotation of the Humerus
Arm should rest easily on the table without pulling the shoulder anterior.

Figure 5-64. Limited Internal Rotation of the Humerus

Note inability of the arm to rotate internally toward horizontal. Concentrate work on the rotator cuff muscles of the posterior shoulder.

In both restrictions, don't forget to work with the teres major and minor muscles, keeping in mind that the teres major is an internal rotator and the teres minor is an external rotator.

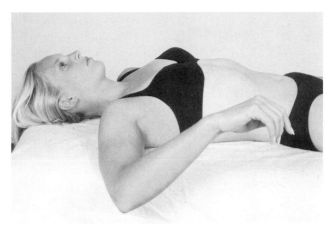

Figure 5-64

Stretching Strategies (DVD 7, 41:09)

Figure 5-65. Pendulum Stretch of the Shoulder Joint

This is one of the easiest and most effective stretches because it counteracts the tension and compression that is a protective mechanism of a sore or frozen shoulder. Clients almost always report improvement of symptoms. Have client protect the back by leaning against a table or chair for support. Let the arm hang loosely with a light weight such as a small soup can and swing the arm in small circles letting gravity be the main force. For this exercise to work properly, it is crucial that the arm hangs very loosely. I often give the image of the trunk of an elephant hanging down. This can be performed many times every day to teach the shoulder to let go of tension.

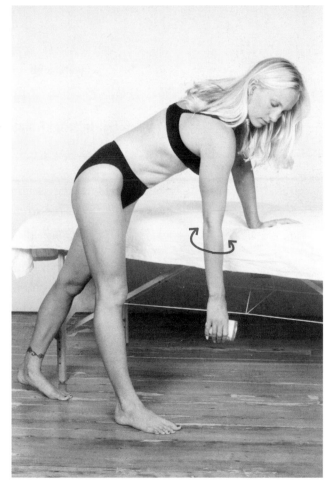

Figure 5-65

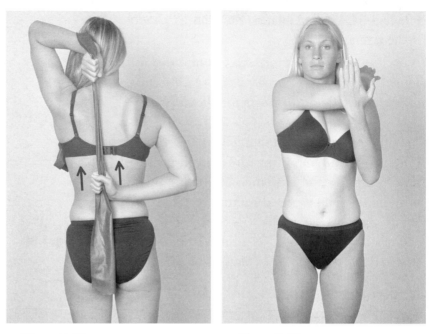

Figure 5-66   Figure 5-67

Figure 5-66. Internal Rotation Stretch of the Shoulder Joint

This exercise is used to increase the ability to internally rotate the bottom arm. Have client grab the band with the lower hand and slowly pull it upward with the other hand. She should not reach up with the lower hand, but let it be passively pulled up. This stretch should not be forced and may take several months to be fully effective in increasing mobility.

Figure 5-67. Posterior Deltoid and Scapula Stretch

Instruct client to slowly pull the arm across the chest and hold for thirty seconds.

PNF Stretches (DVD 6, 08:06)

PNF stretches will be a highly effective tool in your practice for increasing mobility in many joints. It is strongly suggested that you take a workshop to perfect your skills in these techniques. In addition to a PNF stretch for the shoulder, an example of stretching the hamstrings will also be shown to help illustrate the procedure.

Figure 5-68. PNF Stretches for Internal Shoulder Rotation

Anchor the shoulder and then gently move arm down to a relaxed end range of motion. Have the client carefully externally rotate her arm by lifting up against your resistance and holding at the end range for six seconds. Then, have the client take a large breath (you too!) and on the out-breath gently attempt to stretch for an extra degree or two. Do not try to accomplish too much; a small gain is significant. This is very effective in retraining the body as to what an appropriate end range is. This photograph demonstrates stretching into internal rotation, but it is equally effective in the opposite direction to increase external rotation.

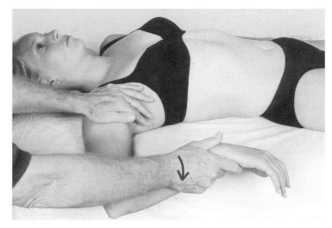

Figure 5-68

Figure 5-69. PNF Stretch for the Hamstrings

The hamstrings are frequently used to demonstrate PNF stretches. With the knee straightened to full extension, stretch the leg to the end range of stretch. Have your client push her leg down against your unyielding resistance for six seconds and then stretch her leg in an upward direction.

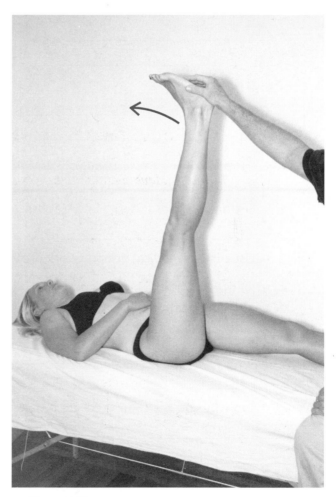

Figure 5-69

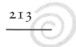

CLIENT INFORMATION

Name _____ Age _____ Sex F ☐ M ☐ Date _____

Referred by _____

Please describe complaints or problem areas _____

_____

_____

_____

Are these a result of injury? If yes, please provide a brief explanation and date of injury.

　　Injury _____ Date _____

Prior Treatment _____

_____

_____

Surgeries:

　　_____ Date _____

　　_____ Date _____

　　_____ Date _____

Medical Information:

　　List medications I should know about _____

　　_____

　　List current medical or body work professionals you are seeing _____

　　_____

Exercise & recreational activities:　　　　　　　　　　　　Frequency:

_____ _____

_____ _____

_____ _____

Explain why you are coming for treatment and what you hope to achieve _____

_____

_____

_____

SYMPTOMS

Please indicate areas of discomfort on diagram using marks listed below to indicate degree and type.

X   Slight pain

XX   Moderate pain

XXX   Severe pain

Y   Numbness

Z   Stiffness or Immobility

Other pertinent Information _____

_____

_____

I am aware that I am responsible for payment if I cancel appointments with less than 24 hours' notice.

Signature_____ Date _____

Client information is confidential. I encourage you to ask questions about any procedures I am performing or to communicate with me freely about anything that you experience either during or after a session.

DOCTOR'S LIEN

To: Attorney _____

_____

_____

Doctor:

Re: Reports and Doctor's Lien

I do hereby authorize the above Doctor to furnish you, my attorney, with a full report of his examination, diagnosis, treatment, prognosis, etc., of myself in regard to the accident in which I was involved.

I hereby authorize and direct you, my attorney, to pay directly to said Doctor such sums as may be due and owing him for medical service rendered me both by reason of this accident and by reason of any other bills that are due his office and to withhold such sums from any settlement, judgment or verdict as may be necessary to adequately protect said Doctor. And hereby further give a lien on my case to said Doctor against any and all proceeds of any settlement, judgment or verdict which may be paid to you, my attorney, or myself as the result of the injuries for which I have been treated or injuries in connection therewith.

I fully understand that I am directly and fully responsible to said Doctor for all medical bills submitted by him for service rendered me and that this agreement is made solely for said Doctor's additional protection and in consideration of his awaiting payment. And I further understand that such payment is not contingent on any settlement, judgment or verdict by which I may eventually recover said fee.

Dated _____ Patient's Signature _____

The undersigned being attorneys of record for the above patient does hereby agree to observe all the terms of the above and agrees to withhold such sums for any settlement, judgment or verdict as may be necessary to adequately protect said Doctor above named.

Dated _____ Attorney's Signature _____

Attorney: Please date, sign and return one copy to Doctor's office at once.
　　　　　Reply envelope attached.
　　　　　Keep one copy for your records.

BILLING TEMPLATE

Mary Brown
CMT
1234 Fifth Street
Des Moines, CA 94618
(555) 123-4567
SS# 123-45-6789 (or Tax ID Number)

Patient:
Joe Smith
9876 Fifth Street
Oakland, IA 50310

Date	Description	Charges	Payments
1/2/07	Diagnosis: 847.1 (Thoracic Strain) 97140 Manual therapy to upper thoracic and cervical area for injuries sustained in auto accident on 12/17/06—60 minutes	$120.00	0
1/9/07	(Alternative billing possibility) 97123 Massage to cervical area 15 minutes Additional 15 minutes	 25.00 25.00	
	97140 Manual Therapy to upper thoracic 15 minutes Additional 15 minutes	 30.00 30.00	 0

Total Charges	$230.00
Payments	.00
Balance Due	$230.00

Chapter Six

Planning Your Session

Establishing a Strategy for Your Session

How do you plan a strategy for working with your clients? Is your massage a chess game with only two moves? Are your major decisions about whether to begin with clients lying face down or face up? To begin work on their backs or their legs? Those are fairly simple decisions, but as your techniques become more sophisticated, the decisions about how to a plan a strategy become more complex as you make crucial decisions about how to best spend your time.

Once you are extricated from the restraints of having to give equal attention to all parts of the entire body in one session, you will have the freedom—and the responsibility—of deciding which areas of the body will benefit from thorough and focused work. You may still want to give a full-body massage, but you might spent the greater part of the massage on one or two areas, while performing quick energetic work on the rest of the body.

Students who begin to work with focus on a few key areas invariably report that they find the work more rewarding and fun as they begin to give more significant and lasting benefits to their clients. Clients call to report significant changes in posture, holding patterns, or resolution of pain. The profound changes they experience prompt them to make regular appointments for bodywork as an essential element of their health care rather than as an occasional gift to themselves.

It may not be as easy as it sounds to make the transition from full-body massage to localized work. There is security in a fixed sequence of strokes that are essentially the same for all clients. However, most of us have had the experience of receiving bodywork from someone who magically seems to know where the core of our particular tension resides. Rarely is anyone born with this talent. It does take time to develop the skill of knowing where to focus, but persevering through the awkward stage of experimentation with localized work will enable you to reap great rewards.

To formulate a plan for each individual, some sort of criteria are necessary to evaluate where your clients hold stress. Different people have different methods of determining this. It is certainly helpful to rely on verbal cues from our clients, but it is important to remember that pain may be the only criterion that our clients use. Often pain is the response of a vulnerable area to tightness elsewhere. Some therapists are adept at discerning psychological or energetic cues. Some are masters at visually analyzing tension, while others have amazing tactile sensitivity. Most of us are better at one or two of these and have a tendency to rely on the skills we are most confident using.

The problem with limiting yourself to one of these skills is that different clients will present different cues; some may be energetic, while others are visual. The greater the arsenal of evaluative tools at your disposal, the better you will be at knowing where to direct your attention. It is fun to expand our skills based upon our areas of strength and confidence. If, like myself, you are stronger in your tactile abilities than, for example, your visual skills, test yourself by trying to use your less developed senses to analyze the holding patterns of a client. Then verify your analysis by using a skill in which you have more confidence. For example, attempt to analyze stress patterns by utilizing your vision even if you are not confident in that ability. Then corroborate your findings using your touch. You will find that your skills in other evaluative techniques will quickly grow.

The subject of *bodyreading* is far too complex to be covered in depth in this text. It is best learned by observing real people as they move, rather than static pictures. It is a talent that should be a life-long pursuit for serious bodyworkers. Many of the increasingly numerous structural schools offer theories of bodyreading as a basis for their techniques. If you are interested in broadening and refining your skills in this subject, take a workshop or two that focus on evaluating stress in bodies. It is advisable to get an eclectic view by studying with different teachers who may specialize in a particular discipline such as Rolfing®, Hellerwork, Feldenkrais®, Somatics, Traeger®, or Alexander work.

There are numerous other philosophies to explore, so don't feel limited to studying only with a disciple of the better known theories; excellent practitioners who don't fall under a label may have just as much to offer.

The following sections will cover some broad topics to consider when evaluating your clients for patterns of stress.

Primary and Secondary Tightness

Just because a client complains of a tight or painful muscle, it may not be the wisest strategy immediately to dive in to soften that particular muscle. Some muscles are tight or in spasm because they are overworked as they attempt to counter the effects of tight antagonist muscles that your client may not be aware of. It is important to determine if tightness is a *primary* or a *secondary* reaction.

A common example would be the rhomboids, which can be in spasm as they attempt to counteract the effects of a tight chest or shoulders that roll inward. Softening or stretching the rhomboids without first lengthening the anterior chest muscles may even exacerbate the problem. I once worked on a professional violinist who had been told that he needed surgery for constant pain in his midthoracic spine. Everyone who had treated him spent time attempting to soften the spasms in his mid-back without success. Instead of treating the painful area, I spent thirty minutes opening his left anterior shoulder and chest, which were rotated inward from a lifetime of holding a violin to his chin. His rhomboids on the left side were then able to relax in their battle with the front of his body, and the rhomboids on the right side were also able to relax in their competition with the muscles on the left side of the spine. With this strategy, the pain immediately subsided without even being massaged, while if I had stretched his rhomboids, it would have only provided temporary relief or might have exacerbated his problem by moving him deeper into his pattern of anterior shortness.

Most of us have experienced the phenomenon of having a client complain of pain on one side of the spine or neck, only to find that the opposite side is much tighter. The important goal in such cases is to attempt to introduce balance into the body so muscles do not have to compete with each other in a tug of war.

The following are a few examples of secondary tightness that are a response to the primary stimulus of a stronger antagonist muscle.

- Anterior tibia or shin splints, which are overworked in response to tight calf muscles.

- Posterior neck muscles responding to tight scalenes or vice versa.

- Tight hamstrings attempting to counteract either short and tight quadriceps or tight lumbar fascia.

- Internal rotators of the leg and groin, which are working to counteract tight external rotators.

- Rotator cuff tightness, which is responding to tight chest muscles.

A Short and Tight Muscle Versus a Long and Tight Muscle

In most cases a tight muscle is a short muscle, but this is not always the case. This is in some ways related to the primary versus secondary shortness example in the preceding section but has some subtle differences. Let us take the example of the rhomboids that are painful because of the fatigue of countering tight anterior chest muscles that are pulling the shoulders forward. If the client is successful in pulling his scapulae together from the back, the rhomboids would be *short* and tight. If the chest were winning the battle so that the shoulders were pulled forward and the scapulae were pulled wide apart, then the rhomboids would be *long* and tight in their losing battle. The rhomboids would be painful in both cases; however, the strategy for working this area would be different for each case. If the rhomboids were short, you would consider stretching them to return the shoulder girdle to a more neutral position. If they were long and tight, you would still work to soften them and increase circulation in the area, but would emphasize lengthening the muscles attached to the lateral scapula and the chest area so that the rhomboids could relax.

The hamstrings are another muscle group that can be tight in either a shortened or lengthened position. In both cases, clients will complain of tightness and may not realize that the solution is more complex than just stretching the hamstrings.

Figure 6-1. Long and Tight Hamstrings

In this case, the hamstrings are tight and long. The anterior tilt of the pelvis has pulled the ischial tuberosities up, which puts a stretch on the hamstrings. They will be tight in their losing battle attempting to pull the pelvis down into a neutral position. Stretching the hamstrings would not be productive. Working to lengthen the rectus femoris, which is pulling down on the anterior pelvis, softening the lumbar fascia to allow the crest of the ilium to drop down, or releasing the psoas muscles, which are pulling the lumbars forward, all might be useful strategies to restore balance to the pelvis and reduce the strain to the hamstrings.

Figure 6-2. Short and Tight Hamstrings

The hamstrings are tight and short in this case. They are pulling the pelvis into a posterior tilt. You would probably want to emphasize stretching them to allow the pelvis to move to a more anterior tilt, or to lengthen the abdominal muscles, which are pulling up on the pubic symphysis.

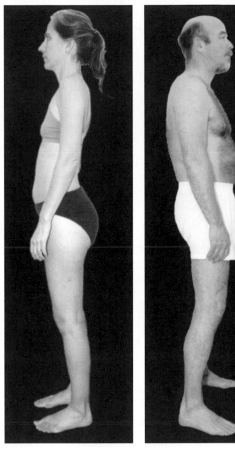

Figure 6-1   **Figure 6-2**

Bodyreading

THE LAST TWO PHOTOGRAPHIC EXAMPLES provide a transition to the subject of bodyreading. As mentioned earlier, the subject is much too complex to cover in depth in this manual and is best studied with live subjects. If you find the following discussion interesting, many massage schools offer classes on the subject and many of the "structural integration" disciplines have their own unique philosophies. To whet your appetite, a few basic approaches will be offered here.

The purpose of bodyreading is to help you design a strategy for working with your client. Most of us read the posture of our clients at an intuitive level even if we are not aware of it. With conscious awareness and practice, this skill can be based upon consistent quantifiable standards that will free you from the "shotgun" approach of working the entire body equally in hopes of finding core areas of tension. Let us look at some simplified examples while remembering that most people are complex and sometimes conflicting blends of the following generalizations.

Front-to-Back Balance

As a general rule, the flexor muscles lie on the anterior aspect of the body, while the extensor muscles lie on the dorsal aspect. Ideally, these two groups are in balance with each other so a person can stand erect with a minimum of effort. However, for many people, one group dominates.

Figure-6-3. Flexor Dominant Posture Pattern

Most of the tightness, especially in the hip flexors and in the thorax and arms, lies in the front of the body. Notice how the angle of the elbow betrays tension in the biceps (flexors), and how the abdomen and chest are pulling the upper body forward. The anterior neck is short and the head is pulled forward.

Clients exhibiting such posture will often complain of pain in the posterior aspects of their body as the overworked extensor muscles attempt to counter the strain imposed by the muscles on the front of the body. The lower thoracic back will be tight and painful in its efforts to hold the spine upright.

Remembering the section of primary versus secondary shortness, a good strategy should consider spending more time on the primary shortness in the front of the body by releasing the hip flexors, freeing the ribs to rise, and opening the front of the neck. This would provide more relief than focusing all the attention on the muscles that are complaining in the back of the body.

Figure 6-4. Extensor-Dominant Posture Pattern

Here, the extensors are dominating the posture; they are short and tight. While the chest and abdomen are open, the posterior muscles show the most strain. The angle at the elbow is straight and the triceps are tight and pulling the humerus back. The thorax is tilted upwards from the front as the lower thoracic muscles pull it down from the back. The neck shows strain from being pulled too far back.

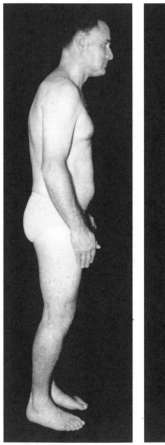
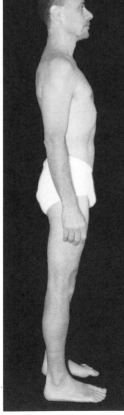

Figure 6-3   **Figure 6-4**

In this case, minimal work would need to be done on the front of the body. Putting the client into side-lying position in a C-Curve or fetal position would lengthen the posterior muscles such as the erector spinae while you work on them.

Figure 6-5. C-Curve

Working in a position to stretch the lumbar fascia and turn the pelvis under will both lengthen the low back and give a cue to your client to let the pelvis fall in the rear.

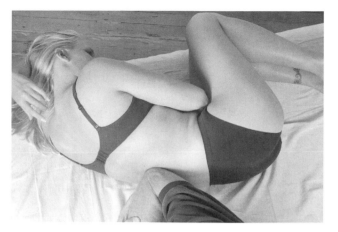

Figure 6-5

Side-to-Side Balance

Figure 6-6. Side-to-Side Balance

At first glance, the side-to-side strain patterns are more easily discernable. The right shoulder is high and the spine is curved or bent to the left. When given this example, many students immediately jump to the conclusion that the right trapezius is lifting the shoulder and that softening and lengthening that muscle will return balance to the body.

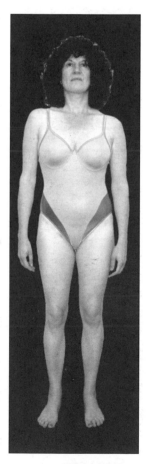

⊚ Before proceeding further, it is very important to clarify the distinction between a **functional** and a **structural** imbalance. A functional pattern of postural imbalance is usually caused by some activity or habit. In the above example, a high right shoulder might be a pattern from lifting the right shoulder to carry a purse or to hold a telephone to the ear while writing, or as a compensatory pattern from an old shoulder injury. A structural pattern is more complex. It may come from osseous conditions such as a scoliosis that is rotating and bending the spine to the left. If this were the case, softening the right trapezius would have little effect because the shoulder is resting on ribs that are rotated up because of the side-bending of the spine. Another structural cause could be a previously broken clavicle that is short and pulling on the shoulder.

Because of the complexity of structural patterns such as scoliosis, the bodyreading examples here will focus upon functional issues resulting from short muscles. These conditions are much more responsive to Deep Tissue Massage.

Figure 6-6

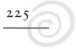

In planning a strategy to work with the high right shoulder resulting from functional causes, the main decision would be whether the right shoulder is pulled up by a short and tight trapezius and levator scapula muscle, or if the left side of the body is short in the trunk area. Also consider whether a short quadratus lumborum or psoas muscle on the left side is bending the spine to the left so that the right shoulder is simply resting on ribs that are rotated upwards.

Internal Versus External Patterns

Viewed from the front, some people appear to be rotated *out* from the anterior midline, while others appear to be pulled inward in the hips and chest area. The following photographs demonstrate a consistent or congruent pattern in both the thorax and legs. In reality, many people will have differences between their upper and lower bodies that may result in twisting patterns such as one forward shoulder or hip. A strategy for this pattern would need to be more complex.

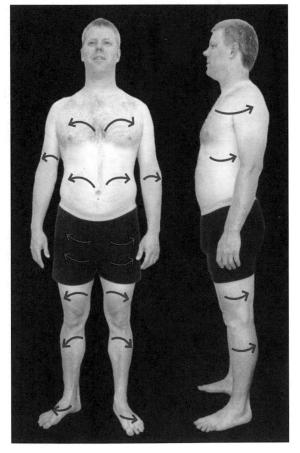

Figure 6-7. External Rotation Posture Pattern

Imagine the body as being composed of two cylinders continuing up from the feet to the shoulders. In this case, the cylinders would be rotated outward as the arrows demonstrate. The arms are pulled back and the chest is open without exhibiting the upward tilt of the thorax that was shown in the extensor-dominated example (Figure 6-4). The pelvis is flared wide in the front, and the legs are rotated outwards so that the feet point out at a forty-five degree angle.

A strategy for this client might focus on releasing the external rotators at the hips, working to lengthen the back muscles such as the rhomboids from the midline in a lateral direction, and lengthening the rotator cuff muscles so the arms can relax inward.

Figure 6-7

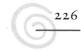

Figure 6-8. Internal Rotation Posture Pattern

Again using the cylinder analogy, notice how the body rotates inward towards the anterior midline. The arms are rotated inwards and the chest is tight. The adductors in the legs are dominating the external rotators in the hips, the pelvis is narrow in the front, and the feet are turned slightly inward.

This pattern indicates need for more work in the front of the body, particularly in the chest area, the anterior deltoid, and the latissimus dorsi and lateral scapula. Placing your client in side-lying position with the leg extended down to release the tensor fascia latae from the front, and to free the lateral scapula would be effective strategies. Releasing the iliacus muscles could also help widen the pelvis from the front.

Figures 6-9 a and b. Freeing the Lateral Scapula

These techniques demonstrate a method of educating your client to release a habitual postural pattern. Allowing the scapulae to move more medially will open the chest and bring the arms back.

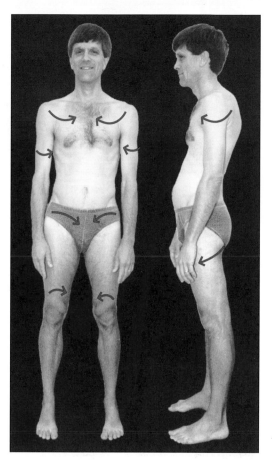

Figure 6-8

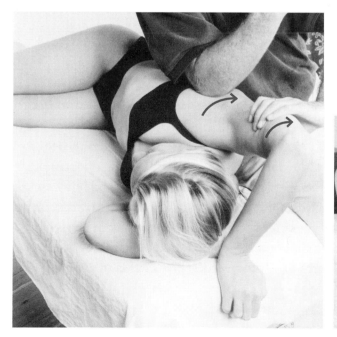

Figure 6-9a

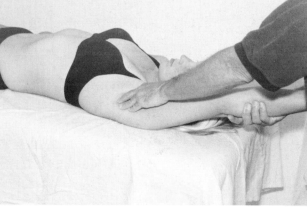

Figure 6-9b

 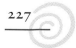

Active Versus Passive Movement

MANY OF THE DIRECTIONS IN THIS BOOK call for *active* instead of *passive* movement of clients when performing strokes. This means, for example, that if you were lengthening the tibialis anterior muscle, you would ask your client to plantarflex her foot while performing the stroke. This maneuver is usually more effective than the two alternatives of just having the ankle remain in a neutral position (no movement) or of your manipulating the foot with your other hand (passive movement). Active movement offers you the chance to see and feel restrictions to smooth movement. Does the foot invert or evert when asked to plantarflex, and how far can it move on its own? Once patterns are determined, you may give instructions to "point your foot straight as you extend it," or "pull your heel back as you point your toes," or other directions, which can help to retrain movement while you are working.

Another advantage of active movement is that it frees your other hand to work when stretching tissue. For example, you could anchor both heads of the gastrocnemius muscle above the knee with each of your hands while you ask your client to flex and extend her knee.

The principle of *reciprocal inhibition* accounts for the third, and perhaps the most important advantage of asking for active movement while you are working. Reciprocal inhibition is actually a simple reflex which enables smooth and easy movement at most joints. When a muscle contracts, its antagonist is inhibited from contraction so the two muscles do not compete against each other. In the example of tibialis anterior muscle, when you ask your client to extend her ankle, the gastrocnemius and soleus muscles contract and send relaxation impulses to their antagonist, the tibialis anterior. This relaxation allows you to actually stretch the muscle while you are working on it. Another example would be asking the client to straighten the knee while massaging the hamstrings. (The contraction of the quadriceps will initiate relaxation of the hamstrings.) A client with tennis elbow could be asked to flex the wrist while you are working to lengthen the muscles that extend the wrist.

There are countless examples of asking for the contraction of an antagonist muscle, but asking for active movement is particularly useful when working with the neck. Instead of leaving the neck in a neutral position or passively moving it with one hand while you are working, try asking for movement. You can have your client rotate or side-bend her head in the opposite direction from the side you are working. This simple principle will enable your client to significantly increase the ability to rotate her neck, as sometimes a tight muscle will relax.

Don't be intimidated by these explanations; you do not need to be a kinesiologist to use these techniques. An easy way to utilize this principle is simply to ask your client to move their joint in a direction that will stretch the muscle you are working on. The antagonist will automatically contract and do your work for you.

Asking for active motion may sound like a radical change from having your client always passively lying on the table while "zoning out," but you will find that many clients who are looking for results will enjoy the chance to participate and appreciate the effectiveness of your work. The transition from passive to active massage is actually not that large a change. Most of the time, your clients will be able to comfortably relax in positions you have always utilized; however, here's hoping you will try some of the postures demonstrated in this book! Asking for movement just once or twice during a massage at an important area is all that is necessary. Once you begin to work this way, it will become easy occasionally to interact with your clients in a more active manner.

Seated Work (DVD 7, 1:10:55 through 1:22:00)

Sometimes our good work can be negated when our client gets off the table and has to function in an upright position. All that work of softening the trapezius muscles will be quickly negated if she walks off into her daily life with her shoulders up to her ears. Seated work is an excellent way of integrating your work so that the client can experience relaxation while erect in gravity rather than lying down. Just a minute or two of seated work on the trapezius and levator scapula muscles can leave a lasting message about how to hold the shoulders. It is also an excellent way of addressing the small complaints some clients have when they have not adjusted to moving again after an extended period on the table.

This work is very different from the *chair massage* that is performed in specially designed massage chairs for the purpose of giving short sessions to clients who are fully dressed. Though you may want to do some quick work to the shoulders when regular clients are fully clothed after the massage, most of the strokes are best performed on skin to facilitate stretching of tissue, and of course you would have your client wearing underclothes while performing this work. Beginning with a little work when they are clothed will educate them on the benefits of the seated position, and allow an easy transition to work when they are wearing underwear.

One drawback to conventional chair massage is that the client remains in a forward flexed position for the entire massage. In seated massage in your private office, you have the advantage of placing your client in many different positions to place muscles in a stretch while working.

A bench will work better than a chair for seated work. It should be high enough that the client's knees will be slightly lower than the pelvis so that the feet can offer support. Except for specific work intended to stretch the spine into flexion, be sure to have your client sitting up straight with a proper lumbar lordosis. This will minimize strain to the lumbar and sacral areas, which are more vulnerable in an upright position.

Seated Trapezius Work

To familiarize yourself with these techniques, begin with seated trapezius and levator scapula work. Even a minute or two of this work is very beneficial, and can be performed when your client is dressed after the massage. Choose a regular client who has the habit of lifting her shoulders in the upright position, and suggest a bonus of a few strokes to that area after a massage. You will quickly have a fan of seated work.

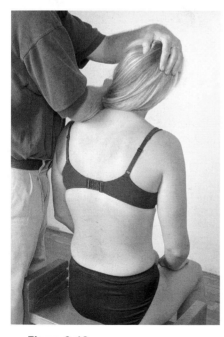

Figure 6-10

Figure 6-10. Seated Trapezius Work

Be sure to have the client sitting erect with a proper lumbar curve. The knees should be lower than the pelvis so that the feet can be used for support. Work on the trapezius can be performed either unilaterally or bilaterally. Working unilaterally offers the advantage of tilting or rotating your client's head with your other hand, or the client can actively tilt or turn her head to the opposite side. Either active or passive stretching of the neck and head away from the side you are working will effectively stretch the trapezius and other upper shoulder muscles. The disadvantage of unilateral work is that uneven stress is placed on the sacrum and spine. Working bilaterally does not allow for as much stretching of the trapezius but is safer for clients who have back problems because force is transmitted evenly down the spine. With both strategies, working in a medial to lateral direction gives a feeling of lengthening and lowering the shoulders.

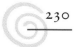

Seated Scapula Work

Figure 6-11. Seated Medial Scapula/Subscapularis Work

When working with your fingers to access the subscapularis muscle, you may want to brace your elbow against your own body to provide leverage as you protract and rotate the scapula with your non-working forearm or hand.

Figures 6-12 a and b. Seated Midthoracic Work

It is often helpful to work with your elbows or knuckles above or medial to the scapula when your client is seated. Postural holding patterns that are not evident when lying down will manifest themselves when your client is erect. This work is especially effective with the trapezius, levator scapulae, and rhomboid muscles. It is important to point out habits of unnecessarily lifting the shoulders or pulling the scapulae together with the rhomboids.

After freeing the scapula, finger, knuckle, or elbow work is very effective in the spinal groove for the entire length of the spine. Allow your client to come up for air occasionally to rest the back and to enable her to feel the benefits.

◎ Notice that even if the head and neck are flexed forward, the low back remains upright in a neutral position.

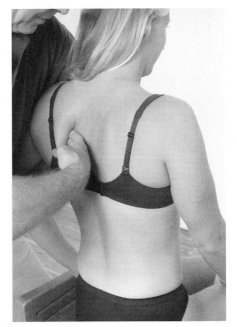

Figure 6-11

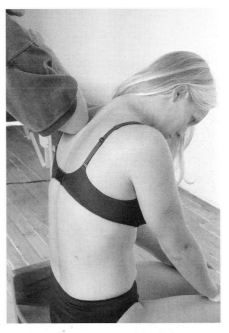

Figure 6-12a

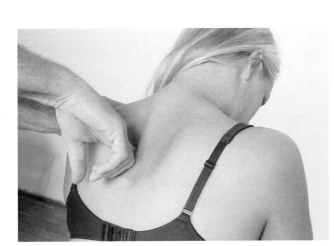

Figure 6-12b

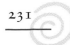

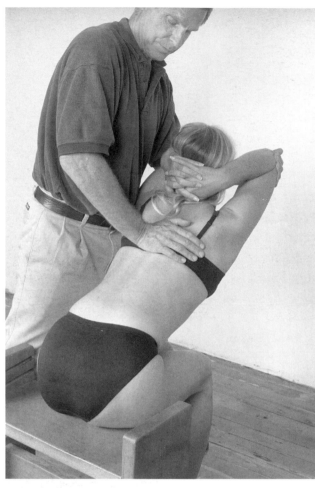

Figure 6-13

Extending the Thoracic Spine

Figure 6-13. Extending the Thoracic Spine

Clients love this position, but be sure to protect your own back. This work can be performed as a broad stretch, or you can use knuckles to perform precise work with the small paraspinal muscles. Slight rocking or side-bending movements can help free immobile vertebrae. For heavier clients, this position can be approximated by sliding the bench back and having your client's elbows resting on the table. Use your right hand as a fulcrum to focus extension at specific vertebrae.

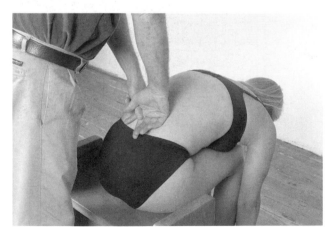

Figure 6-14

Stretching the Lumbar Fascia

Figure 6-14. Stretching the Lumbar Fascia

Have your client bend as far forward as is comfortable. Placing a pillow on the knees or having her support herself with her elbows on the knees are also options. Use broad, spreading strokes rather than applying too much pressure on the lumbars and sacrum.

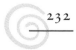

Shoulder Girdle Work

Figures 6-15 a and b. Seated Rotation of the Humerus

This position allows for many possibilities in abduction and rotation of the humerus. Palpate tight muscles and then move the arm into a position that will stretch the muscles while you are working. You will have easy access to the teres and the deltoid muscles.

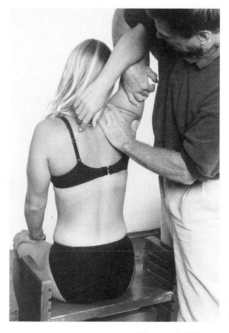

Figure 6-15a

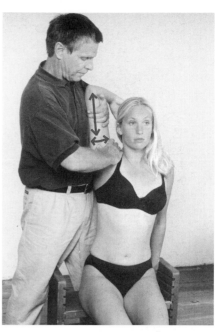

Figure 6-15b

Figure 6-16. Seated Stretching of the Rotator Cuff

Pulling the arm across the chest will stretch the rotator cuff muscles and rhomboids. Experiment with different degrees of arm elevation from chest level to above the head.

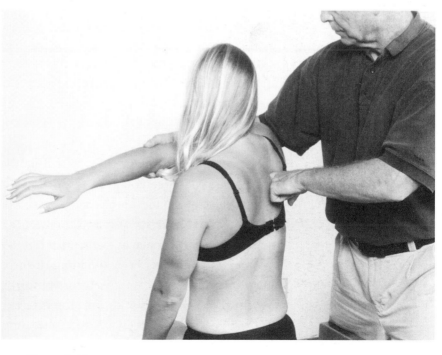

Figure 6-16

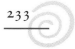

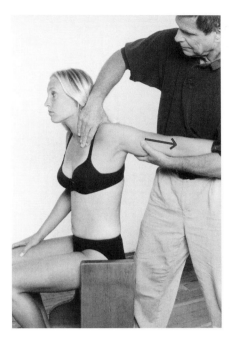

Figure 6-17

Figure 6-17. Seated Opening of the Chest

Support your client's arm with your body rather than just grabbing it with your hand. Work slowly and ask for breath while pulling arm back and anchoring on chest tightness.

Integrating Strokes and Strategies into Your Massage Style

Becoming an accomplished practitioner of Deep Tissue Massage, or of any form of bodywork, involves a thorough understanding of the principles of the work and mastery of the technical aspects. The strokes and strategies demonstrated in this manual should offer a multitude of options to effectively treat specific conditions and areas of the body.

◎ It is important to remember that a stroke that is performed in a mechanistic manner without a clear intention of purpose can become an empty gesture.

I sometimes notice that the focus required to learn the mechanics of new techniques can impart a somewhat impersonal and pedantic style to new students. The performance of strokes can begin to dictate the tone of the massage, rather than the needs of the client dictating the choice of strokes. As important as the techniques demonstrated in this manual are, the nurturing and healing intention behind the massage may still be the most important aspect of the Deep Tissue Massage you are performing. From my ten years of work in a physical therapy center, I am convinced that in addition to the very quantifiable myofascial benefits of massage, the genuine concern for the individual being treated is the magical element that makes our work so effective.

The pendulum has been swinging in the opposite direction from the old reputation of massage as either prostitution or a pampering indulgence to be performed in low lights with burning incense. Sometimes, however, the pendulum will swing too far in the other direction before settling in its final position. Requirements for continuing education and certification now emphasize the more scientific and medical aspects of training. Lately, I have heard several therapists denigrating "feel good" or relaxing massage as outdated and ineffective. As I sample the different massage therapies, I sometimes experience an ambiance that resembles the coldness of a doctor's office.

A woman friend who became an attorney over twenty years ago laughs at how she and her women friends initially attempted to be accepted by the male dominated law profession by denying their femininity. They dressed in somber suits, wore neckties, and even bought "wing tip" shoes in their attempts for acceptance. Thankfully, this practice was short-lived.

The complaints and symptoms that our clients present to us are rarely simply the result of a tight muscle or two that can be magically remedied by a fancy or esoteric technique. I suspect that massage therapists will be in great demand long after robots are designed to mimic massage strokes. Emotions of fear, sadness or depression, anger, or isolation can create or be created by the tension or pain in the body. It is important for massage therapists to carefully examine how they would like to practice their profession and to not be intimidated into donning the white medical coat and stethoscope if it conflicts with their personality, goals, and style of massage.

The next chapter addresses your ability of self-expression through your individual skills and the type of massage practice you would like to experience. The acquisition of highly effective techniques in no way needs to conflict with your expression of who you are. Your skill in the technical aspects of Deep Tissue massage can be an additional tool in the expression of your caring and healing nature.

Chapter Seven

Fulfillment Through a Thriving Practice

NTERING THE BODYWORK PROFESSION CAN INVOLVE A CIRCUITOUS PATH. If, when I was in graduate school studying exercise physiology twenty-five years ago someone had described the life and satisfaction I have with my work now, I would never have thought it possible. In all truth, not a day goes by that I don't feel extraordinarily lucky, as I occasionally glance through my windows at the trees outside my quiet office, doing work I love with people I deeply care for. Although someday in the future I may work only a few easy days a week, I look forward to continuing my work as long as I am physically able.

Fulfillment has different meanings for different people. For some massage therapists, it may be the freedom to work part-time in order to devote more time and energy to one's family, artistic interests, or travel. For some it may be the close and loving relationships with regular clients. For others, the possibility of earning a very good income while doing rewarding work is a major goal. As long as you retain a fresh and enthusiastic attitude in your work, it really is not important if you work with two or twenty clients a week. However, it is important to be able to work on as many clients as you desire. I have known excellent massage therapists who feel unfulfilled because they are unable to generate enough business to feel successful.

One of the joys of teaching bodywork is the satisfaction of hearing how some students have transformed their businesses from tenuous day to day hopes for appointments into thriving practices with waiting lists. Not only are they busier, but by honing their skills and continuing to expand their knowledge, they find their work more interesting, fun, and fulfilling. I would love to have all my students achieve this, but unfortunately, I am also saddened when I see excellent therapists who, like the tree falling in the forest with no one there to hear it, have difficulty establishing and maintaining a thriving practice. Over the years, I have spent considerable time speaking with therapists and other teachers attempting to deduce the reasons for this. Following, are some of the patterns for success and some of the pitfalls of establishing a fulfilling practice that have emerged from these discussions.

Moving Forward with Your Knowledge

ALTHOUGH THERAPISTS ALWAYS SEEM to leave continuing education workshops with bright-eyed enthusiasm, translating the new knowledge into practice often runs head-on with established work patterns and sometimes with previous training. A large component of learning is not just adding new information, but the letting go of early training or old habits that are no longer applicable as one learns more. Beginning massage training is limited in the amount of detail that can be presented in a short time to inexperienced students. Some people fail to continue to pursue more depth in their understanding of anatomy, working with more powerful tools, or addressing the medical complaints encountered in a massage practice. They continue to give essentially the same massage, albeit with more finesse, that they gave right out of school. Probably the biggest obstacle is to overcome some of the limiting definitions of what constitutes a massage—primarily the idea that in every session the entire body must be covered or the client will walk out without integration or feeling that something has been left out. It is, indeed, a bit frightening to first escape from these shackles, but virtually every therapist I discuss this issue with says that their clients love the special attention to areas needing more work, even if some areas receive only superficial coverage. To utilize new and powerful bodywork training, it will probably be necessary to sacrifice routines that are not as productive. Of course you can also begin to schedule longer sessions to allow detailed and specialized work within the context of a full-body massage.

Time Management

The easiest way to begin providing more detailed work is to clarify your use of time and to exclude superfluous and time-wasting work. Every stroke should have a purpose, and rote, stroke-oriented routines should be eliminated. I repeat my earlier statement that a stroke without purpose can be an empty gesture.

Knowing Where to Work: The most useful skill is to know where to work to give the most benefit to your client. Master bodyworkers rarely need sophisticated tricks or routines; they simply go to where the work is needed. This is a skill that is quickly learned as you choose two or three issues that will help your client leave the session with new feelings of freedom or lack of pain. Don't try to accomplish too much and, rather than spreading yourself too thin, be satisfied with concentrating on only a few areas that will leave your client feeling more whole. Quick integration work in the other areas near the end of your session can be remarkably effective without spending a great deal of time.

Knowing When to Stop: If knowing where to work is the most important skill, then knowing when to stop working an area may be the next. This skill can be divided into two categories:

Knowing When You Have Accomplished Your Goal: One of the most frustrating aspects of a massage can be when the therapist has relaxed a tense area but continues to work away as if the area is still problematic. In addition to wasting time, this habit can actually create imbalance in the body and give the message that you are giving a rote routine without really tuning in to the client's needs. Become sensitive to the "melt" of muscle and the release of holding patterns, and move on when the work is complete.

Knowing When to Throw in the Towel: Equally frustrating to the client is the case when the therapist continues to work for a long and often painful amount of time on an area that is not ready to release. Sometimes therapists will continue to apply increasingly intense pressure in hopes of winning a battle with a recalcitrant muscle. This not only wastes time, but can leave the client bruised and with lingering discomfort or increased symptoms. If four or five minutes of work on an isolated area does not produce improvement, then it is doubtful that more of the same kind of work will succeed just because you are pushing harder. You should either attempt a new strategy or let discretion be the better part of valor and move on. It may be that some other area must first release for this area to relax. It is also possible that the area may let go the next day when it is ready, if you have provided careful and focused integrative work or released a primary strain pattern elsewhere that is initiating the compensatory tightness.

Working at the Proper Depth: Early massage trainings need to instill caution in new students until they learn how to safely penetrate through superficial tissue or to properly prepare an area for work. However, these early caveats are often carried to extremes so that therapists spend undue time lightly "warming up" tissue with ineffective light work or working on relaxed superficial tissue instead of sinking to deeper areas of tension. Some clients describe this overly careful approach as similar to having an itch that someone is tickling instead of scratching, or even scratching in the wrong place. One of the most important skills you can have for deep tissue work is to as quickly as possible sink into and work at the depth where resistance is felt. This skill will not only help with your management of time, but will impress your clients with your skill at honing in on problem areas.

⊚ One of the most important skills you can have for deep tissue work is to as quickly as possible sink into and work at the depth where resistance if felt.

Other Pitfalls That Limit Growth

From years of teaching, I encounter several major misconceptions that keep therapists from evolving their practice into more effective and rewarding work.

Fear of Disturbing your Client by Changing Positioning: Early training emphasizes the quiet relaxation of clients over therapeutic goals. Most everyone must overcome the hesitancy to instruct clients to move to positions that afford more effective treatment options. Having clients move to the side-lying position, sliding down so that feet can hang over the end of the table, removing the head rest in the prone position so that it is possible to work with the spine in rotation and side-bending all offer dramatic possibilities for treatment that far override the discomfiture that we feel in asking the client to move. You will find that clients are very open to movement when they feel the benefits that different positions offer for work.

Draping: Moving limbs, turning into side-lying, or having clients actually sit up for more detailed work such as shown in the previous chapter may create draping difficulties. Draping is a functional skill and not an art form. I find that lack of confidence in draping is one of the biggest factors preventing therapists from trying more innovative techniques and strategies. I once had a student write to thank me for "... freeing me from the obsession of excessive draping concerns at the expense of sacrificing function in my work." Of course you must take care of your clients' modesty concerns, but having extra pillows, towels or other props, and sometimes just explaining that you need to use some positions that make draping a bit awkward will allow you to accomplish many expanded goals. Many experienced therapists simply ask clients to wear underwear that can be worked around when the situation requires it.

Early Caveats: Many early warnings in massage training persist beyond their usefulness, instilling in therapists a trepidation in expanding their work or creating a tentative and timid style of work. I encounter long-time therapists whose fear—of working on the anterior neck, working near the spine or mobilizing joints (including vertebrae), the abdomen, or gluteal area—prevents them from growth. Of course you should not work any area unless you feel safe doing so, but very often this hesitancy is based upon lack of anatomical knowledge rather than prudence. Other therapists deprive their clients of the benefits of decompressing joints by always working in the direction of venous return to the heart. It is often advisable to work in a distal direction if you can give the client the feeling of decompressing a joint such as at the shoulder, femur, or other areas where you can work in the direction of muscle lengthening.

Lactic Acid Myths: I am amazed at the persistence of the urban legend that lactic acid can remain trapped in muscles in a solid form that is released in massage and therefore causes post-massage pain. This misconception is difficult to dispel because no scientists even consider it worth debunking because they never encounter such misinformation among their peers. In reality, lactic acid is only in the muscles in substantial amount for a maximum of 30 to 60 minutes following anaerobic exercise and metabolized from the Krebs cycle into pyruvate as a source of energy. The importance of this misconception is that some therapists work too hard and bruise tissue and then rationalize the improper work by this myth or the "no pain, no gain" adage.

Lubrication: Most therapists use entirely too much or the wrong kind of lubrication. Probably the biggest distinction between relaxation massage and deep tissue or myofascial work is the focus on grabbing and stretching tissue rather than gliding over it. It is crucial to use very little lubrication (lotions are often better than oil); consider using a product that is more of the consistency of shoe polish and has a beeswax base.

The "Horse" Stance: Many teachers are bewildered by the persistence of some students in using this stance, where the knees are significantly bent, the pelvis is tucked under and both feet are parallel to the body. You should lean into your stroke with your body weight, so that horizontal force is provided by your legs, with one leg behind to provide the force. When properly using your weight rather than muscular effort, if your hands were suddenly pulled out, you would actually fall on the client. The Horse Stance is an excellent martial arts posture for grounding energy through the feet, but ineffective for deep tissue work since it makes the utilization of gravity transmitted through the arms virtually impossible. Without use of your body weight, it will be necessary to "muscle" your strokes, which will not feel good to your client and will predispose you to injury from straining.

Elbows and Knuckles Are Used Only for Deep Work: These tools are simply effective ways of working with tissue and are perfectly appropriate for gentle work when they provide mechanical advantage over other tools. With just a little practice, your elbow can be almost as sensitive as your fingers.

Just as the original information of early training may be no longer applicable to your skills or even incorrect, new information may also be inappropriate or incorrect as well. The important thing is to separate the information from your affinity for your teachers and to not persist in unproductive patterns simply out of loyalty to any teacher. Observe any education for its broad truth and also for its applicability to your own individual needs.

The Realities of Entering the Bodywork Profession

Practical Matters

The choice of the word "profession" instead of "business" is intentional. For some, the realities of providing income to live require initial focus on the business aspects and postponing the lofty aspirations of a profession. Beginning a massage practice is hard work and requires skills that may have little to do with your massage expertise. For instance, it is necessary to reach well beyond your friends for a client base.

Many new therapists begin their practice by working in a spa, chiropractor's office, or similar setting. This is an excellent way to gain the experience of working on many different people to hone the skills you learned in school. There are no worries about establishing an office, recruiting clients, and paying for the initial expenses of beginning a business. Spas provide a relatively consistent income, and sometimes offer health insurance, vacations, and free membership to the facilities. There is also the advantage of the camaraderie of working with a group of like-minded friends.

On the other side of the coin, such work may have aspects that prevent the transition to a more lucrative and rewarding private practice. The biggest danger is that of "burnout." Rarely do I see therapists continue working in a spa setting for over five years. Obviously, the therapist only receives a percentage of what the client pays. It is necessary to work on approximately twice the number of clients to earn your target income. In order to make a satisfactory living, many therapists overwork and become injured and disenchanted as they struggle for survival like characters in a Charles Dickens novel.

One other concern about working for someone else is that it can severely limit your opportunities to express your individuality. In a spa or chiropractor's office, the clientele for the most part dictate what type of massage you will give. When you have your own private practice, this relationship is reversed. Your personal style and expertise will quickly bring you the clients you want to work with in the manner you choose.

Obviously, as much as I recommend working in a spa or chiropractic setting to initially expand your massage skills, I have strong opinions about the advantages of working for yourself in the long run. These feelings come from the elation I see in massage therapists who make the transition to working in their own practice. Many therapists feel trapped by their dependence on their spa income and find it difficult to make the transition to working for themselves. They are working full time and don't have the time or energy to suddenly make the leap to wean themselves from their spa or chiropractor's job. There are no simple answers to this conundrum.

Everyone must find their own answer, but the following suggestions have proved helpful. The first step is to envision the type of massage practice you would like to have and choose a realistic time frame to achieve this incrementally. Without clarity of purpose, things rarely develop on their own. Most therapists do not have the reserve of money to tide them over until their practice is busy—this is the reason most got into working for someone else in the first place. It is necessary to face the fears about temporarily sacrificing some income, but it should be kept in mind that a sudden transition is not necessary, and perhaps not ideal. Initially, many therapists set aside one day a week to only promote their business and work on private clients. If they aren't booked for the day, they spend the time on networking and promotion. As they slowly build their practices, they substitute more days for private work until they can support themselves.

One big expense of having your own practice is setting up an office. For that reason, out-call massage is a very practical alternative and way to work on your own until you have enough private clients to cover the expense of maintaining an office. A private office is the ideal solution for many, but many massage therapists who choose to not work at home are unable to commit to renting a full time office space. Consider getting together with several of your peers to rent an office together and work out a schedule to share the space. As your client load grows, you can add time at the office.

As mentioned at the beginning of this section, there are many advantages to working for someone else; it may be exactly what you envision for yourself. However, if you aspire to having your own clients, please spend the time and energy to achieve this goal. You may find that as a result you consider yourself to have a profession rather than a job.

Self-Esteem

Most of us need to feel that we are trying to be the best that we can be—with growth comes confidence. One of the most interesting phenomena that I have encountered both in my own continuing education efforts and that I see in my students is the sudden, often miraculous upturn in business after taking a class teaching new skills. Invariably, after a class, students call to report that they suddenly have new clients appearing out of nowhere. It is hoped that students acquire new skills in classes that make them better massage therapists, but I am quite sure that the increased confidence and self-esteem that accompany this learning are also large factors in attracting clients. Yet many therapists rarely take continuing education classes.

Sometimes the obstacles to growth and learning can be internal mind-sets rather than a lack of interest. Instead of a sense of complacency, it seems that many new massage therapists are a bit intimidated by climbing back on the horse of learning. The difficulties of beginning a massage practice can take a toll on one's confidence and energy. It can be a frightening experience to step out of one's comfort zone to face the sometimes intimidating prospect of learning that there is room for improvement in our work. The years of competition in our school system have conditioned many of us to look at classes as an anxiety-generating test of our skill and knowledge rather than as a vehicle for growth.

Imagine that you are considering buying stock in a company and find that it has not allocated any money for "research and development." Would you make an investment in such a shortsighted company? Some massage therapists do exactly that in making no commitment to expand their expertise while expecting their practice to be successful. Your initial education, whether a 150-hour training or a 1000-hour certification program, can only start you on the path to success. Bodywork is an incremental learning process and can best be learned while practicing out in the real world. There are 1000-hour programs that give a wealth of information to students who are not yet prepared to assimilate or integrate the subtleties of the information. Such a situation is a bit like taking tennis lessons for years before actually playing a game. You will be amazed at the power of learning new skills and how continuing education provides a boost to your self-esteem and enthusiasm.

Distinguishing Yourself

To have a successful practice, we face tremendous competition, not only from the medical profession and other healers, but also from our colleagues. One of the keys to a successful and fulfilling practice is to differentiate yourself from the growing number of other massage therapists out there. Ideally you can do this by being "better" than your competition, but "better" is quite subjective and not a guarantee of success. What it takes to differentiate yourself from those practicing generic massage is not so much to be better, but to be *different*. To be different, you need to cultivate specific skills that will distinguish you from the masses, meaning not just taking classes, but applying what you've learned.

So often, I see students leaving class excited with their new knowledge and full of high hopes for positive change in their professional lives. They may have a better sense of the layers of the body and how to utilize different tools to enable them to work more deeply and effectively. They are able to work with less effort and more sensitivity and are less injury-prone. They are able to give a much better massage, but for some, this does not translate to a busier practice.

For years I was puzzled about why this occurred for some students, while others reported immediate and dramatic improvements in their ability to recruit new clients by word-of-mouth, which they attributed to their improved skills.

It finally became clear that the students who reported dramatic increases in business were actually working differently with their new techniques. They were asking clients to turn on their sides for work; they were working with bony articulations to increase mobility of joints; they were working with more slow strokes. Most importantly, they escaped from the "beat the clock" treadmill of attempting to give equal attention to the entire body in one short session or to treat every client the same.

While still performing their regular full-body massages, these therapists began focusing on two or three different areas that needed extra care in each massage. Their clients immediately noticed the difference in their work and began to get more regular work and to refer friends. Many reported clients commenting, "I've never had a massage like that before." Before long, the practitioners had reached a critical mass where regular clients and their referrals were keeping them booked in advance.

So what about those therapists whose new skills seemed to have little impact upon their busyness? It became clear that most of these students, even if they became much better at massage, did very little different in their work. Many expressed a hesitancy or resistance to ask clients to actively participate in the massage process by moving into different positions. They never asked clients to actively move limbs in order to retrain muscular movement patterns, or never slowed down to free up vertebrae or ribs that were not moving freely. They continued to attempt to work with equal attention to the entire body, neglecting core areas of tension because of a feeling of urgency to complete the massage.

Most importantly, these therapists continued to give basically the same massage, albeit better, that they had always given. Most expressed a fear of using the new tools they had learned because they were locked into an inflexible perception of what a massage should be. Based upon a model they learned in their first massage class, they sabotaged themselves by projecting this view of what a full-body massage should be onto their clients. They feared that their clients would think that their "new" massage was strange and different rather than having the trust that clients would appreciate their new skills and ways of working.

◎ Basically they were sabotaging themselves by worrying about being "different" when that is exactly what they needed to do to elevate and distinguish themselves from all the other massage therapists who are giving essentially the same massage.

Fulfillment Through Self-Expression

SEVERAL TIMES THROUGHOUT THIS MANUAL, I have mentioned the importance of being creative in your work—of escaping from the "cookie cutter," or "paint by the numbers," massage. It is an unusual individual who thrives in a job of mindless repetition or stifled creativity. If you hope to retain a fresh and optimistic enthusiasm in your work, it is essential to feel that you are giving your clients the gift of your best skills tailored to satisfy their needs.

Whether in art, music, sport, work, or our relations with our fellow men and women, one of the joys of life is the ability to express the unique individual we are. Just as an articulate person may only use a small portion of her vocabulary to express herself, you may use a limited number of the strokes demonstrated here. However, one only needs read great poetry to grasp the power of concise, articulate, and well-chosen words. In the same way, judicious use of the strokes and techniques shown in this manual may help you to better convey a deep message to your clients. Just as having the vocabulary to communicate clearly enables better writing, it is hoped that the strokes and techniques demonstrated in this manual will be helpful in adding to the vocabulary and language through which you express yourself in massage and thus, add to the fulfillment you receive from your work.

Suggested Reading

General Bodywork

Chaitow, Leon. *Muscle Energy Techniques with CD-ROM.* 3rd ed. Oxford, England: Churchill Livingstone, 2006. ISBN-10: 0443101140, ISBN-13: 978-0443101144, 276 pages, $79.95 USD.

   This comprehensive text describes the theory and practice of Muscle Energy Techniques (MET). It demonstrates manipulative techniques in which a patient, upon direction from the therapist, actively moves limbs against a distinct counterforce applied by the practitioner. These techniques are combined with other treatments in physical therapy, osteopathy, chiropractic, and manual medicine. This is an excellent book, not only for the techniques that are demonstrated, but also for the understanding of kinesiology.

Chaitow, Leon, Graeme Chambers, and Viola M. Frymann. *Palpation and Assessment Skills.* 2nd ed. Oxford, England: Churchill Livingstone, 2003. ISBN-10: 0443072183, ISBN-13: 978-0443072185, 400 pages, $71.95 USD.

   This is an excellent guide for palpation and assessment of muscular and skeletal dysfunction.

Clay, James H., and David M. Pounds. *Basic Clinical Massage Therapy: Integrating Anatomy and Treatment.* LWW Massage Therapy & Bodywork Series. Philadelphia: Lippincott Williams & Wilkins, 2002. ISBN-10: 0683306537, ISBN-13: 978-0781756778, 450 pages, $52.52 USD.

   The clear pictures of anatomy and overlays of therapists' hands during treatment make this a very accessible text for classroom or private use. It is very comprehensive in information for specific clinical techniques such as compression, stripping, myofascial, and cross fiber strokes.

Dalton, Erik. *Advanced Myoskeletal Techniques.* Oklahoma City: Freedom from Pain Institute, 2005. ISBN-10: 1599752883, ISBN-13: 978-1599752884, 315 pages, $87.95 USD.

This is an incredibly detailed and useful book that tackles extremely interesting and difficult subjects, not only of specific bodywork techniques, but more importantly, giving an understanding of how the body works. This enables the student to do so much more than just mimicking strokes and allows that next level of understanding that can actually facilitate healing.

Davies, Clair, Amber Davies, and David G. Simons. *The Trigger Point Therapy Workbook: Your Self-Treatment Guide for Pain Relief.* 2nd ed. Oakland, CA: New Harbinger Publications, 2004. ISBN-10: 1572243759, ISBN-13: 978-1572243750, 323 pages, $19.95 USD.

This is another of the classics of bodywork, both for therapists and as self-help for clients, for a wide variety of complaints. It is clearly written and comprehensible to laypeople, but also very useful for therapists, either for treatment or education of their clients.

Hendrickson, Thomas. *Massage for Orthopedic Conditions.* Philadelphia: Lippincott Williams & Wilkins, 2002. ISBN-10: 078172287X, ISBN-13: 978-0781722872, 550 pages, $50.95 USD.

This is an excellent reference of manual medicine that also is applicable for massage if the practitioner is knowledgeable about anatomy. The text describes specific conditions, assessments, and protocols for treatment.

Juhan, Deane. *Job's Body: A Handbook for Bodywork.* 3rd ed. Barrytown, NY: Station Hill Press, 2002. ISBN-10: 1581770995, ISBN-13: 978-1581770995, 488 pages, $39.95 USD.

This could be considered the granddaddy of bodywork education books, both for practitioners and the general public. Not a "how-to" book, it is rich with philosophy, but also with well-documented science from cell biology to neurophysiology and physics. An excellent book for understanding the mind as well as the body and how they interrelate.

Lowe, Whitney. *Orthopedic Assessment in Massage Therapy.* Daviau-Scott, 2006, ISBN-10: 0-966119630, ISBN-13: 978-0966119633, 305 pages, $39.95 USD.

This is another highly recommended text with a broad range of information about assessing injuries and troubleshooting issues with your clients, as well as treatment suggestions—an excellent book for a wide range of bodyworkers.

McIntosh, Nina, and Mari Gayati Stein. *The Educated Heart: Professional Guidelines for Massage Therapists, Bodyworkers and Movement Teachers.* Reprint ed. Philadelphia: Lippincott Williams & Wilkins Publishers, 2003. ISBN-10: 0781748860, ISBN-13: 978-0781748865, 248 pages, $26.95 USD.

This thorough but down-home and unpretentious overview of the professional and ethical issues of a bodywork practice not only gives important practical information about how to have clear boundaries with your clients, but is also fun to read. Many client/practitioner problems could be prevented if any therapist were to read this invaluable resource for both students and experienced practitioners.

Myers, Thomas W. *Anatomy Trains: Myofascial Meridians for Manual and Movement Therapists.* Reissue ed. Forewords by Leon Chaitow and Deane Juhan. Oxford, England: Churchill Livingstone, 2001. ISBN-10: 0443063516, ISBN-13: 978-0443063510, 278 pages, $52.95 USD.

This is another of the true innovations of bodywork that has transformed the way countless people work by explaining the role of fascia in creating strain patterns in the body. Unlike some other books, which attempt to simplify structural bodywork and give scripted routines, Myers offers a deeper understanding that can be applied in many settings. It is indispensable to the understanding of holistic treatment of the forces that disrupt the balance of the body, enabling the treatment of causes rather than just of symptoms. It should be in everyone's library, regardless of the specific type of bodywork practiced.

Rolf, Ida P. *Rolfing: Reestablishing the Natural Alignment and Structural Integration of the Human Body for Vitality and Well-Being.* Revised edition. Rochester, VT: Healing Arts Press, 1989. ISBN-10: 0892813350, ISBN-13: 978-0892813353, 304 pages, $24.95 USD.

Along with *Job's Body* and *Awareness Through Movement* this book was a groundbreaker and true classic of the bodywork movement. Ida Rolf goes to considerable effort to not disclose her specific treatment plans, but the information about fascial anatomy and postural stress is applicable to any body worker. It is worth having in your library just for the historical value.

Simons, David G., Janet G. Travell, Lois S. Simons, and Barbara D. Cummings. *Travell & Simons' Myofascial Pain and Dysfunction: The Trigger Point Manual.* 2nd ed. Philadelphia: Lippincott Williams & Wilkins, 1999. ISBN-10: 0683307711, ISBN-13: 978-0683307719, 1664 pages, $194.95 USD.

This is an updated version of the classic trigger point encyclopedia, and so much more than that. Its information may be too detailed for general use, but any serious trigger point therapist should have this as a reference if Claire Davies' text leaves you wanting more information. The anatomy drawings are worth the price of admission.

Stanborough, Michael. *Direct Release Myofascial Technique: An Illustrated Guide for Practitioners.* spiral bound ed. Oxford, England: Churchill Livingstone, 2004. ISBN-10: 0443073902, ISBN-13: 978-0443073908, 232 pages, $49.95 USD.

This is an in-depth and easy-to-understand book that is extremely accessible in its explanations of the causes and treatment for most conditions encountered in a bodywork practice. It is very well illustrated with numerous photographs. Unlike many such books, it also covers postural issues with clear instructions on how to provide balance to the body as well as just treating complaints.

Spinal Mobilization

Greenman, Philip E. *Principles of Manual Medicine.* 3rd ed. Philadelphia: Lippincott Williams & Wilkins, 2003. ISBN-10: 0781741874, ISBN-13: 978-0781741873, 700 pages, $99.00 USD.

The skill of understanding the workings of vertebrae can transform your practice and open all sorts of new visions. This book is serious medicine and is another classic, but it is suggested that you try to find a copy to view before deciding if it is appropriate for your practice. It provides detailed and clear explanations of spinal mechanics and specific treatment options.

Maitland, Jeffrey, and Kelley Kirkpatrick. *Spinal Manipulation Made Simple: A Manual of Soft Tissue Techniques.* Berkeley, CA: North Atlantic Books, 2001. ISBN-10: 1556433522, ISBN-13: 978-1556433528, 164 pages, $20.00 USD.

By giving a distilled view of Greenman's more extensive text on the same subject, this book can best be described as an unintimidating guide to working with bones and ligaments. It provides an understanding of spinal mechanics as well as clear, less-detailed descriptions for mobilization of joints.

Self-help Books for Clients of Exercise Instruction

Chatz, Mary Pullig. *Back Care Basics: A Doctor's Gentle Yoga Program for Back and Neck Pain Relief.* Berkeley, CA: Rodmell Press, 1992. ISBN-10: 0962713821, ISBN-13: 978-0962713828, 264 pages, $21.95 USD.

This is an excellent book to have several copies of to loan out to clients. Being able to provide excellent information for self-care is extremely helpful to your practice, either by instructing clients yourself in safe and effective stretches or by steering someone into a new understanding of their body by having them explore yoga or other self-help options. This book provides excellent maintenance suggestions as well as safe and effective ideas for specific back and neck problems.

Feldenkrais, Moshe. *Awareness Through Movement: Easy-to-Do Health Exercises to Improve Your Posture, Vision, Imagination, and Personal Awareness.* Reprint ed. San Francisco: HarperSanFrancisco, 1991. ISBN-10: 0062503227, ISBN-13: 978-0062503220, 192 pages, $14.95 USD.

This famous book is designed for self-help for your clients, but specific exercises can be demonstrated to your clients in your practice. These exercises are extremely worthwhile and effective, but many people find them difficult to perform alone and opt to work with a Feldenkrais practitioner.

Johnson, Jim, and Scott D. Boden. *The Multifidus Back Pain Solution: Simple Exercises That Target the Muscles That Count.* Oakland, CA: New Harbinger Publications, 2002. ISBN-10: 1572242787, ISBN-13: 978-1572242784, 132 pages, $12.95 USD.

This book provides an understanding of the muscular component of back pain that will prove worthwhile for therapists, but is primarily intended for the general population as instruction for self-treatment. An excellent resource to keep for loans or sale to clients.

McKenzie, Robin A. *Treat Your Own Back.* 6th ed. Orthopedic Physical Therapy Product, 2006. ISBN-10: 0958269238, ISBN-13: 978-0958269230, 72 pages, $10.00 USD.

McKenzie, Robin A. *Treat Your Own Neck.* 3rd ed. Orthopedic Physical Therapy Product, 1997. ISBN-10: 0473002094, ISBN-13: 978-0473002091, 63 pages, $10.00 USD.

As important as bodywork is to alleviate back and neck pain, giving clients the empowerment to help themselves is a profound gift. Both of these books are excellent for patient self-help. The newer editions cover in more detail the anatomical rationale for the exercises. These books have helped thousands of people conquer serious back or neck problems.

Anatomy and Physiology

Acland, Robert. *Acland's Video Atlas of Human Anatomy.* Philadelphia: Lippincott Williams & Wilkins, 2003. ISBN-10: 0781743575, ISBN-13: 978-0781743570, 7-DVD Set, $159.95.

If you can't take a dissection class, then this is the answer. In fact, viewing this collection will probably give you more of an understanding than most college-level anatomy classes. Some of the more detailed brain or nervous system anatomy may be beyond many therapists' interest and the individual DVDs are available separately, but the set is nicely packaged and a real bargain that can be viewed over and over with added understanding gained each time.

Biel, Andrew R., and Robin Dorn. *Trail Guide to the Body: How to Locate Muscles, Bones, and More.* 3rd ed. Boulder, CO: Books of Discovery, 2005. ISBN-10: 0965853454, ISBN-13: 978-0965853453, 420 pages, $52.95 USD.

This acclaimed book is excellent to either learn anatomy or as a review with palpation guides for precision in treatment. It offers excellent illustrations, combines bodywork ideas implicit in the anatomy information, and makes the study of anatomy both interesting and fun. The author also offers many other products such as flash cards and other books.

McMinn, R. M. H., R. T. Hutchings, J. Pedington, and P. H. Abrahams. *Color Atlas of Human Anatomy.* Reprint edition. St. Louis, MO: Mosby-Year Book, 1993. ISBN-10: 0815158513, ISBN-13: 978-0815158516, 368 pages, $46 USD.

Having exquisite dissection and photographs, this is my favorite anatomy atlas. Almost as good as having your own cadaver, it will increase anyone's understanding of the body—including your clients'. My clients always are amazed and grateful when I show them the anatomical structures I am working on, and I've had several over the years be so interested that they purchased the book for themselves.

Netter, Frank H. *Atlas of Human Anatomy.* 3rd ed. Oxford, England: W. B. Saunders, 2002. ISBN-10: 1929007116, ISBN-13: 978-1416033851, 612 pages, $72.95 USD.

This is a wonderful anatomy atlas for medical study, clinical reference, and patient education. Not only is it an excellent text, but is also timeless and true art with its beautiful hand-drawn illustrations. You will keep this book forever.

Powers, Scott K., and Edward T. Howley. *Exercise Physiology: Theory and Application to Fitness and Performance.* 6th ed. New York: McGraw-Hill Humanities/Social Sciences/Languages, 2006. ISBN-10: 0073028630, ISBN-13: 978-0072878653, 624 pages, $92.50 USD.

Although this text is written for serious students of exercise physiology, it is not overwhelming for bodyworkers. Massage training often neglects the "why" of how bodies function, with primary emphasis upon the anatomy. Actually many other physiology book are excellent, but having an exercise focus, this book gives the therapist who works with athletes some added insights into the issues they present.

Index

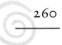

About the Author

Art Riggs is a Certified Advanced Rolfer® and massage therapist who has been

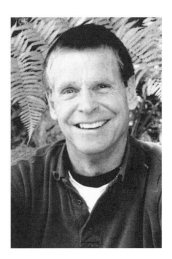

teaching bodywork since 1988. A lifetime of hard physical activity and high level athletic pursuits including ultra-marathons led him to bodywork, first as a grateful recipient, and later as a student. The fulfillment he experienced in both receiving and performing bodywork led him away from his graduate studies in Exercise Physiology at the University of California, Berkeley to a full time career as a Rolfer and teacher of Deep Tissue Massage. He has conducted numerous workshops for health spas and for medical professionals, including physical therapists, and has assisted in Rolf Institute trainings.

For the first ten years of his practice, Riggs specialized in myofascial release at a physical therapy clinic where an interest in the treatment of injuries was cultivated. He has worked with several Olympic athletes, professional football and basketball players, and professional dancers and musicians to treat injuries and to improve performance. However, his teaching and the practice of working with the general population to provide a better awareness of their bodies and allow more ease and comfort in their everyday lives remains the most gratifying aspect of his work.

Riggs lives and teaches in the San Francisco Bay Area. For more information please visit www.deeptissuemassagemanual.com.

DEEP TISSUE MASSAGE AND MYOFASCIAL RELEASE

The 7-volume companion DVD set for *Deep Tissue Massage: A Visual Guide to Techniques* is a very useful expansion of the techniques presented in this book. Seeing them performed in real time with full explanations gives an in-depth understanding of working at different depths, speed of strokes, and the subjective qualities of touch that are impossible to convey with still photographs.

Nearly *11 hours* of demonstrations, treatment plans, and instruction will transform the way you work and show you how to approach virtually every situation encountered in a bodywork practice.

"I wish I had had this resource 12 years ago when I was in physical therapy school. The book and videos have dramatically improved the quality of my work and saved my body from injury."

Patrick Hannum
Physical therapist and Rolfer

"'Deep Tissue Massage and Myofascial Release' has enabled our school to plan a 100 hour Deep Tissue curriculum around its clear progression from the basic skills to clearly defined strategies."

Julie Morrison
Director of Massage, Western Career College, Pleasant Hill, CA

DVDs 1 & 2 — FUNDAMENTALS OF DEEP TISSUE MASSAGE AND MYOFASCIAL RELEASE

Approximately 3 hours of easy-to-understand and immediately accessible techniques:
- Working with different layers of the body
- Biomechanics for more efficient use of your energy and prevention of injuries
- Tools—proper use of Fingers, Knuckles, Fist, Forearm and Elbow
- Specific strokes to add precision and a goal-oriented approach to solving problems and providing mobility and ease of movement for your clients

DVDs 3, 4 & 5 — PROTOCOLS AND STRATEGIES

4½ hours of specific plans to cover the whole body including:
- Working with proper functioning of joints through alignment of soft tissue
- Spinal mechanics and joint mobilization
- Specific protocols for working with the Feet, Legs, Pelvis, Psoas, Back, Rotator Cuff, Cervicals, Arms, Cranium, and much more

Deep Tissue Massage and Myofascial Release: A Video Guide to Techniques is applicable for:

- Massage students wishing to expand their relaxation-based practices to include structural and more therapeutic emphasis
- Teachers or schools looking for a well-defined curriculum to greatly improve your educational tools
- Experienced bodyworkers looking to expand your skills and add new and fun ways to rejuvenate your practice

DVDs 6 & 7 — TROUBLESHOOTING (Treatment Plans For The Most Common Injuries And Complaints):

Approximately 3 hours of instruction to enable you to work with confidence treating:

- Plantar Fasciaitis and Achilles Tendonitis
- Knee, Back, Hip, and Neck restrictions
- Rotator Cuff problems
- Overuse injuries to the Arm, Wrist, and Thoracic Outlet
- PNF Stretches and other tools to expand your efficacy and make your work more fun

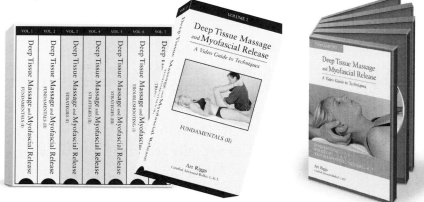

"The thorough demonstrations—not only of specific techniques, but the subtleties of working with tissue—show how to work with virtually all soft tissue situations encountered in a bodywork practice. Art Riggs has made this valuable information accessible for both the relatively new therapist and experienced professionals performing sophisticated clinical therapy."

Helen James
Masters in Physical Therapy, Stanford University & Professor Emeritus California State University, Fresno

". . . so much more than just showing strokes. This series has transformed the way that I work. At a fraction of the price I'd pay at a school, this video is an entire bodywork course that I can study at home. It will be a reference for years to come"

Justine Jacobs
Massage Therapist

*Please visit our website at **deeptissuemassagemanual.com** for more details and how to order the videos at the lowest price available. This manual may also be ordered at a substantial discount with further reductions for larger orders.*